11 REASONS WHY YOUR BACK ACHES— AND WHAT YOU CAN DO ABOUT IT

1. **TRAUMA**—sudden twisting, strain, improper sitting, other injuries
2. **BAD POSTURE AND CURVATURE**
3. **"SLIPPED DISC"**
4. **CONGENITAL AND DEVELOPMENTAL DEFECTS**
5. **INFECTIONS AND TUMORS**
6. **ARTHRITIS**
7. **SYSTEMIC DISEASES**—can be caused by vitamin deficiencies
8. **AGING AND HORMONAL CHANGE**
9. **PREGNANCY**
10. **REFERRED PAIN**—originating in other areas of the body
11. **STRESS, FATIGUE, AND TENSION**

ONCE AND FOR ALL—RID YOUR-SELF OF AGONIZING BACK PAIN! THIS IS THE ONE BOOK THAT SHOWS YOU HOW TO GET RELIEF —SIMPLY AND FOREVER!

Oh, My Aching Back

Oh, My Aching Back

*A doctor's guide to your back
pain and how to control it*

by Leon Root, M.D.
& Thomas Kiernan

*Introduction by Dr. James Nicholas
Director of Orthopedic Surgery at Lenox
Hill Hospital, New York City, and
personal physician to the Jets*

Illustrated by William Thackeray

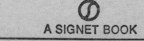

A SIGNET BOOK

NEW AMERICAN LIBRARY

Authors' Note

Although this book is the result of a full and complete collaboration between the two authors, it is written in the first person singular voice of Dr. Root so as to spare the reader confusion of identities.

L.R.
T.K.

Introduction

by Dr. James Nicholas

Director of Orthopedic Surgery at Lenox Hill Hospital, New York City, and personal physician to the Jets

It is a pleasure to write an introduction for a book that is clear, concise, and accurate, and which is at the same time accessible to the layman. Dr. Root is experienced in the treatment of pain and his book deals with an affliction of man which, at times, has influenced the course of history. Backache has been with the human race since man assumed an erect position. People from all walks of life are afflicted, ranging from presidents and great athletes to workers and growing children. There are untold numbers of individuals suffering from backache. It is a poorly understood condition leading to a great deal of misinformation, and therefore one that has created a great deal of cultism.

The stress of bachache on a patient, along with the disability, economic loss, and other various related problems are well documented in this book. The cause of such suffering to the productivity of the nation is staggering when one considers the numerous compensation and disability claims, as well as the many hours lost from work and daily living comfort. Draft deferrals during the wars have indicated how large numbers of men were unfit to pass even a simple physical examination. Industrial accidents from congenital backache are an important cause of disability. This book emphasizes the anatomy and structural variations that occur, and which lead to such disabilities. The loss of an individual's own personal physical fitness has not been emphasized enough; the maintenance of strength, endurance, flexibility and agility are the key to enjoying life. Backache is one of the most common deterrents to achieving these goals. The inadequate supply of specialists trained in the diagnosis and treatment of backache, when compared with the large number of individuals afflicted, makes the problem much more difficult. As a result there are so many forms of treatment that patients are confused and seek varying types of cultist approaches, which may or may not have any bearing on the true diagnosis.

This book by Dr. Root and Thomas Kiernan, in simple fashion, will do a great deal to help the public distinguish between the diverse nature of backache as to its causes and its evolution. It should dispel much fear and discourage cultism while directing backache sufferers toward a rational approach to treatment. This book not only deals with future developments, but in simple language it shows how so many causes of backache can occur. It details what type of examination a patient should expect, and the varying causes of backache in the young and the old. The effect of trauma, metabolic changes, and psychological implications of such pain are also dealt with so that the patient can better understand his ailment.

Beyond the diagnosis, the most important treatment of backache has always been, short of surgery, a therapeutic exercise program initiated once the pain has been controlled. This book sets forth a number of exercises, in detailed description with diagrams, which are valuable and approved by most orthopedic surgeons.

All of us in orthopedic surgery recognize that chronic backache is one of the most important of our national health problems and requires continuous medical research directed to its prevention. Once neglected, structural changes occur and it is much more difficult to cure. Certain individuals have a predilection for back pain and they must learn their vulnerabilities so as to prevent the excesses that produce the pain and chronic suffering. Physicians as well as patients should profit because the book deals with some intimate, small, but important details that one should be aware of when backache begins. The emphasis on rest, posture, exercise, support, and an accurate diagnosis are very important. I am confident that Dr. Root has made an important contribution to the lay public in educating it about backache. The book is written in a simple language that presents rather complex details in a simplified but surprisingly accurate manner so that fear is dispelled. It should be stressed, however, for people reading this book, that it is not meant to be a textbook from which one can diagnose the nature of their pain. Individuals with backache should have a competent specialist examine them when the pain occurs, so as to be sure of the diagnosis before treatment is instituted. One cannot, despite the simplicity of this book, categorize all the variables which must be considered in an individual before they undergo treatment. People come in all sizes, shapes, and forms, varying degrees of strength and endurance, and propensity for injury, illness, and occupation, and for this reason an accurate diagnosis must be made by the physician. The authors recognize and stress how an early diagnosis leads to proper management. The case histories are extremely representative, and the causes and treatment of backache, with emphasis on annoying conditions which can cause backache, are important if one is to have some type of cohesive program. Dr. Root also stresses the fact that the neck is a contributor to backache, and therefore, in common low-back syndromes, the upper back must be protected against pain as well. He also recognizes how surgery is indicated under certain conditions; but the most important areas in this book, for the average layman, are individual exercises which tend to strengthen the back and help to relieve frustrating back pain.

This book is an excellent example of how a good, sound, informative medical communication on an intricate subject can be made pleasurable reading for laymen.

Finally, although this book does not represent an in-depth discussion of the various new treatments that are available, it does allude to the potential research and medical treatment that is useful in the small number of cases where surgery is indicated.

Foreword

Two questions should be asked at the outset of this book. One is—what are my reasons for writing it? Why is there a need for a comprehensive book on the subject of back problems for the general public? The other is—what are my qualifications for writing such a book?

Why the book? A recent United States Public Health Service report indicates that an astoundingly large number of adults in the United States—close to seventy million—have experienced at least one episode of severe and prolonged back pain in their lives. Another report from the National Center for Health Statistics indicates that currently more than seven million Americans are being actively treated by doctors for chronic back pain, and that new cases are being added at a rate of almost two million a year. According to this second report, at the rate back pain is spreading, in three years more people will suffer from chronic and recurring back problems than from any other single medical ailment.

After perusing these reports it occurred to me that if we were to consider this ailment a disease, back pain would constitute the most massive epidemic our society has ever had to face.

You have most likely picked up this book because you are one of that vast multitude of backache victims mentioned by the two reports. It is for you, then, that I write.

As a practicing orthopaedic surgeon with years of experience dealing with back problems, I know that the great majority of you *need not* endure the pain and wretchedness, and often the physical debility, you are forced to suffer as a result of your faulty backs. Not if you vow to yourselves, with the help of a detailed and informative guide, to put an end to your pain.

Most of your problems are due in the first place to ignorance and mismanagement. The great majority of back ailments that I am required to treat, whether surgically or by other therapeutic means, could have been avoided at the very beginning through the application of a little practical knowledge and common sense when the first ache or spasm manifested itself.

Unfortunately, the very people who will rush their cars off to the mechanic at the first sign of an ineffective shock absorber or sagging spring will not be as faithful to themselves after their first episode of back pain. Aye, as Shakespeare might have punned, there's the rub!

Back ailments are not usually associated with mortality statistics, as is the case with such other major medical problems as cancer and heart disease. Nevertheless I have seen all too often how that first single episode of back pain leads to a lifetime of agony for the victim. As a doctor I am aware not only of the numbers and statistics relating to back disease, but also of the havoc that chronic back pain wreaks in the lives of those unfortunate enough to experience it.

It is an unhappy fact of life that back pain *does* tend to become chronic, and can often turn into a torturous and disabling ailment. I am not trying to scare you, as those of you who have suffered back ailments in their more acute forms will attest.

It is my belief that if people were aware of the most common causes of back pain they would in a large majority of cases be able to prevent its occurrence. In the case of those tens of millions of you who already live under its yoke, with a little knowledge to go along with your motivation you can not only prevent its recurrence but you can forestall the more serious complications likely to arise if it is ignored.

It is not enough that doctors are available for treatment. Treatment is only one side of the backache coin. Doctors are usually consulted only when the pain and other symptoms have progressed to a point where they are no longer indicative of a simple problem, such as strain or poor posture. As Mr. Shakespeare had Cassius say (you will discover among other things in this book that I am quite fond of the famous Bard), "The fault, dear Brutus, is not in the stars, but in ourselves that we are underlings."

The problems that cause back pain can in most cases be solved *before* the pain brings you to your knees with the more severe and costly complications that result when the original signs are ignored. All it takes is a little knowledge and a resolute application of that knowledge—not only on the part of the doctor, but on your part as well. Indeed—

even more importantly on your part, since you are the one who has to live with your back.

There is no need for us to remain underlings to the agony and debility to which our backs are capable of enslaving us. A comprehensive, straightforward, information-packed guide—devoid of tricks and cute writing and promises of quick or magic cures—should be available to victims and potential victims of back pain, so that they may understand their back ailments and learn how to prevent them from becoming a continuing problem in their lives.

This book is such a guide. In the pages that follow I shall explain, in the simplest terms practicable, the general spectrum of back problems. I shall discuss their causes, diagnoses and treatments. More important, I shall discuss what *you* can do to control and prevent the recurrence of *your* particular ailment.

You will note as we go along that the emphasis in this book is on "you." Although not every ailment discussed will be immediately relevant to your particular problem, you will certainly discover yourself in these pages—or perhaps I should say you will discover your back. Of course in one sense, if you have an existing ailment—whether you've just had your first episode of back pain or have suffered for years—everything in the book should be of interest to you. Why? Because in the final analysis this is a book about you and your back. There is never enough you can know about either of these ingenious, however often maddening, creatures.

Now, what qualifies me to write this book? I have already mentioned that as an orthopaedic surgeon I am called upon to treat a great many people with back pain.

When a patient comes into my examining room, all bent over, face twisted with pain, with the words, "Oh, Doctor, my aching back! Can you help me?" I respond with a mixture of sympathy and irony. Sympathy—because I well understand the pain the patient is enduring and how this pain will, more likely than not, become an integral part of his life. Irony—because in so many cases the pain and debility need not have occurred at all had the patient possessed even a rudimentary knowledge of his or her back.

Further irony still—because I know I will be required, in the course of my treatment, to give the patient a detailed lesson on the back and a satisfactory explanation of how the problem came about, to be inevitably answered by:

"Whew, I never realized my back was such a complicated structure—I wish I had known this before."

As usual, people are only interested in learning about their bodies *after* the onset of some affliction. Then, of course, they become experts on that part of their anatomy affected by their ailment. How often have you visited friends recuperating in the hospital who proudly and confidently, with much new-found expertise in medical jargon, provide you with vivid and exhaustive descriptions of exactly what it was that ailed them?

And yet further irony still—because no matter how strongly I emphasize the proper healing and preventive maintenance programs for the problem in question, I know that nine times out of ten, once the initial pain and other symptoms are relieved, the patient will invariably become lax in his or her desire to prevent recurrence and will again begin to take his back for granted. That is, until the next episode, when he will reappear in my office, pale and worn down by the pain, tilted awkwardly to one side, an excruciating grimace searing his face, and say, "Gee, Doc [for now we are on more familiar terms], it came back!"

But don't, as the man said, get me wrong. I'm not being superior, and I'm not putting any of you down. I realize that there's nothing more boring than having to listen to a sermonizer. It is very much a part of human nature to ignore a back problem when the pain and other symptoms are not actively expressing themselves.

I know this only too well because for many years I, too, suffered from chronic back pain. I am, you might say, case history number one. It was not until one particularly painful and disabling episode that I came to my senses and resolved to do something about my back before I was forever thrown into slavery to it. And I did.

Today the memory of the pain and discomfort I used to experience remains strong. It serves as a stark reminder whenever I am tempted, whether out of laziness or my preoccupation with other tasks, to relax my resolve to keep my back in proper condition.

"Proper condition." That's what this book is, in the end, all about. That is the secret of controlling your back problem—keeping your back in proper condition. There are no short cuts and no quick and easy cures.

The memory of my back pain experiences, and the daily program I follow to prevent recurrence, provide probably my best qualification for writing this book. I write not only with the knowledge and experience of a physician who is a specialist in this field, but also with the empathy of one who has, like you, lived with back pain and understands the nature of the beast.

I licked my back problem. Well, perhaps that is an exaggeration. It might be better to say that I tamed it. I got it under control. I think you can do the same, and that's the primary reason for this book.

Another reason is this: because of the press of time, your doctor cannot sit down and discuss your back and its hygiene with you in the detail that you require. Furthermore, you are liable to be nervous and in some pain when you visit your doctor and not likely to remember many of the things he tells you about your back problem. Hopefully, this book will fill in the gaps in your knowledge and help speed you on your way to a healthy, pain-free back.

With these explanations, I give you *Oh, My Aching Back*.

Contents

PART III—THE CONTROL OF BACK PAIN

Part I

The Anatomy of Back Pain

1.

You,
Your Back and
Your Back Pain

If Shakespeare had shared some of his good friends' interest in medicine, he might have composed a sonnet, forgetting the rhyme, which began

> Was there ever a man or lady who
> In a lifetime of endeavour
> Never once experienced the tortures
> Of spasms and pain in the lower back?

After all, Shakespeare was so astute in his appreciation of human nature that he must have been aware of the prevalence of this disorder.

I can count on the fingers of one hand all the people with whom I am acquainted who never once in their lives had a backache. You may rightly wonder why it is that so many of us have back pain. Is it possible that we are all doing something wrong?

In Part II, I will present a more detailed discussion of the causes of back pain, but right now I think it would be useful and pertinent to establish a concept of what the back is and what it does.

Man is a vertebrate, which means that he has a backbone, or spine. The spine has a number of important functions in man's existence, not the least of which is the role it plays as the basis and core of the back.

One of the most devastating things you can say about a person is to call him spineless. By this you intend to convey the notion that he is cowardly, weak-willed, and altogether lacking in admirable qualities. In short, to be without a spine is to be positively sub-human, for the spine is one of the most important attributes of a human being, figuratively as well as literally.

But the physical spine does not exist in a vacuum. Associated with it are nerves, muscles, bones, ligaments, blood and other fluids, fibers, skin.

Of all the components that go to make up the back, the most vital is the spinal cord, which traverses almost the entire length of the spine. The spinal cord is like the telephone cable in an office building that carries hundreds of circuits from a main switchboard to all the offices in the building. Instead of telephone circuits, the spinal cord carries the nerves that come out of the brain. The nerves leave the spinal cord through small openings along its length and supply all the voluntary or skeletal muscles of the body. These are the muscles that activate the things that we actually control with our minds—lifting a cup of tea to the mouth, for instance.

Thousands of little blood vessels weave their way in and around the entire area. Bones, ligaments, muscles, other fluids—even the skin—play important roles in the vital functioning of the back. You'll note that I use the word "vital" in this context. That's because what I'm talking about here is the function of the back that keeps us, figuratively speaking, alive.

In his early stages of development man walked on all four extremities at once, hands as well as feet. Therefore the spine acted as a suspension bridge from head to pelvis. It was held up by the shoulders and forearms in front and by the hindquarters and pelvis at the rear.

At some time during man's early evolution he became a "biped," that is, he began to stand upright on his rear extremities and walk on two feet. He did this without prior consultation as to whether or not his back would be able to adjust to this new position—whether it could take the strains of the prolonged pressure distributed directly upon its surface; whether it would be able to bend and then resume its straight position without snapping or rupturing important component parts; whether its muscle mass, those muscles which act upon it, would be able to support it in an upright position.

The details of how, why and by what process our backs

got to be the way they are we'll leave to the anthropologists to figure out. What we can say without dispute is that the change in man from quadruped to biped, and the accompanying change in the structure of his back, is the main, if not exclusive, reason for the prevalence of low back pain among human beings. If your problem is one that manifests itself in lower back pain, you now know the *general* cause of it.

We still are in the process of evolution, and our backs are probably changing too, but thus far our back development has not caught up with the rest of our bodies under the influence of man's upright posture. About 95 percent of all so-called "slipped discs" occur in the lower spine, just at the level of or near the sacro-lumbar junction. This area sustains the greatest stresses with both bending and improper posture, whether you are sitting or standing. Keep that in mind until, further along, we get into the more specific causes of lower back pain.

The truth that emerges out of all this is that man's Achilles tendon is not really the cord in his heel, *it is his back!* The back has, for ages, been the weak link in man's physical development. Due to its extraordinarily complicated nature, plus the fact that it has been slower to structurally adjust to man's upright position than other parts of the anatomy, the back is more susceptible to ills than any other bodily component.

Case History Number One—Me

I think you'll probably agree that you don't have to be someone special to get back pain. All you have to do is have a back—and who doesn't?

Back pain is no respecter of person or position in life. The plumber and the priest, the housewife and the topless dancer, the truck driver and the minister of state, the clerk and the forest ranger, the banker and the hobo—they are all susceptible. Doctors too.

Probably the only people who don't get back pain are those famous Indian mystics and fakirs who are able to lie for hours on beds of nails. For them neither pain nor anything else of a troublesome nature have any existence.

But most of us are not mystics and fakirs. For us, back pain is very real, altogether too frequent, profoundly discomforting, and no laughing matter, no matter how hard we try.

One of the most vivid childhood recollections I have of my father is the way he used to go around with his torso tilted over to one side, looking for all the world as though he were trying to do an imitation of a badly listing ship. I can well remember the number of times his back was trussed up in tape or secured in a brace in an effort to provide him with additional support. I also recall that he always seemed to be in a good deal of pain. But I never really appreciated what he was going through until it happened to me.

I was twenty years old at the time and nearing the end of my junior year at college. It was time for that annual rite of spring for any athletically ambitious college student—spring football practice. The weather had just started to change after a long, dismal, New Jersey winter, and although the air was somewhat brisk the sun was bright and growing taller in the sky each day.

The practice session had been going along at a leisurely pace. We were running through a punt-return drill. My assignment was to sprint downfield under the punt, deftly avoid two or three blockers, and make the tackle on the punt receiver. We had practiced this play a dozen times. On this particular occasion it seemed so routine that I ran downfield in a fashion that could only be called casual. It was certainly different from my normal habit of tearing off as fast and ferociously as I could. But as any football player will confirm, there is a certain boredom to practice, especially when it's in the spring and you've been running through the same drill for fifteen or twenty minutes. Besides, I was to be Captain of the team that fall and by this time I was feeling pretty sanguine about the whole thing.

As I approached the punt receiver, trying to divine his intentions, I saw him cut toward the sideline. Instead of making a determined effort to tackle him, I made a lackadaisical lunge at him so that my momentum would carry him out of bounds. At that moment two ambitious freshmen who were trying to earn positions on the team decided to block me. One hit me at the knees from one side while the other simultaneously smashed into me high on the opposite side of my chest. I collapsed with a searing pain across my lower back. I felt, literally, as though I had been torn in half. Under normal circumstances, had I been driving hard, this would not have happened. My body would have been tensed and prepared for such a collision.

The pain lasted for only three or four minutes. Playing

football for many years had enabled me to build up a psychological resistance to pain. This was both good and bad. It was good because it made it possible for me to play in spite of whatever bumps, bruises, cuts, wrenches and strains I suffered. It was bad because it got me to believing that I was invincible, indestructible. The person who believes he or she is indestructible is probably the prime candidate for back problems.

At any rate, after a brief respite I was able to continue with practice. But later that day, after having had a shower and returned to my room to study, I began to experience a renewal of the pain. I found it impossible to sleep that night, and by morning I was in agony with severe spasms across my lower back. When I got out of bed and tried to put my shoes on, I couldn't even reach for them. When I tried to stand up I found myself involuntarily bent over at an almost ninety-degree angle. I remembered my father again and said to myself, "So this is what it's all about."

Sound familiar? Just you wait.

With the passing of a few days the spasms mercifully diminished, the pain subsided, and I was able to resume my normal, not very good, posture. By the time the week was out I had completely forgotten the episode. Which was the worst mistake I could have made.

When the back expresses itself through the medium of pain, I later came to learn, it is telling its owner that it has developed a weakness. Whether the weakness is brought about suddenly and dramatically through a traumatic injury such as mine, or through non-specific, less spectacular development, such as in the case of my father—the back is sending a vitally important message. It is telling its owner that he or she should immediately take steps to compensate for that weakness. Just because the pain may go away after that first episode does not mean that the back has gone away. And whether the manifestation is a specific ache or a twinge, a cramp or a crick, a vague soreness or an excruciating pain—the message is substantially the same: "You'd better tend to me now, before I make your life miserable!"

Unfortunately, all too many of us, myself included, have ignored that first message. We have lived to regret it, haven't we? I know I did.

From that single split-second incident on the practice field in the spring of my twentieth year my back became at once my closest companion and my bitterest enemy. Its presence in my life was continual and unrelenting, and the things it did to me I wouldn't do to my worst enemy.

Hah! you say—your troubles came from a football injury, so what do you expect? Wrong. In the years since, while engaged in the study and practice of orthopaedic surgery, I learned that it doesn't really matter *why* the messages from your back start arriving at your brain. It makes no difference whether the first message arrives by virtue of a traumatic injury, such as in my case, or by virtue of poor posture, of strain, of defect, or even of such a seemingly innocuous event as sleeping in a draft.

The message is the medium, to paraphrase Marshall McLuhan. It says it all. In this case, pain is the message. Unfortunately, as I've said, our tendency is to ignore it once it has ceased bleeping out its little code. That's what I did. If I had known what I know now—well, that's hindsight.

But I did ignore my back until it was too late. My back returned to haunt me with uncanny regularity for fifteen years thereafter, each succeeding episode a little worse than the previous one, until finally it became no longer a nuisance but a disability. It intruded itself so thoroughly on my life that my day-to-day existence became a continual sitting on the edge of my chair waiting for the next attack of pain and contortion. When I wasn't lying in bed, that is.

I literally had to be brought to my knees before I finally grabbed the bull by the horns and resolved to do something about my back. Thankfully, as a result of an intensive program of self-devised preventive therapy, I was able to rebuild my back. I no longer find life an experience of sitting on the chair's edge. I only chastise myself for having waited fifteen years before doing something about my back, doubly so for having ignored the original signs of weakness when I experienced my first episode of pain.

My early introduction to back pain and to the vulnerability and susceptibility of the back not only made me respect the importance of this area to the entire function of man but eventually led to my interest in orthopaedic surgery and to my decision to become a specialist in this field.

The orthopaedic surgeon is carefully and exhaustively trained in the anatomy, physiology and kinesiology (the study of the motion) of all joints and muscles in the body. He must understand the causes of back pain and how the back reacts to it, and must be skilled in the treatment of back problems.

It would be melodramatically false if I were to tell you

that as I lay upon the ground that brisk, fateful spring day I resolved then and there to become an orthopaedic surgeon. But if I knew then what I know now, it most certainly would have been a natural thought to have.

Case History Number Two—You

Do you recall your first episode of back pain? When was it—thirty years ago? Fifteen? Or just last week? Whenever, I would consider it a safe bet that you didn't do much, if anything, about it.

Most likely you shrugged it off, and each succeeding episode as well, until you began to notice that your back was erupting with more frequency and, each successive time, with more pain and discomfort.

By now you were forced to the unhappy conclusion that you had a back problem.

If you were and are like most people, this realization only reinforced your stubbornness, pride and determination—you were not going to let a bad back stand in the way of a free and active life. You would learn to live with it!

And so you did, until a few episodes later when you began to notice that you were walking around with a slight list, or that it was becoming increasingly more difficult to bend over, or that you couldn't sleep, or that certain motions that once came as naturally to you as the gull takes to the air had suddenly deserted you. Or, most perplexing and annoying of all, that your legs were atrophying and that you were unable to walk without a limp, without spears of pain shooting down your thighs.

By this time you might have decided to seek professional help. The likelihood is that if you went to a qualified doctor you received excellent medical advice and treatment. The relative success or failure of the treatment you received depended mainly on two things—how much your back had degenerated, and how willing you were to apply yourself to the measures necessary for proper regeneration and cure.

Ironically—and in many cases tragically—at the beginning there was very little wrong with your back that you couldn't have repaired yourself. The pains you started to get in your back were simply its response to the bad or careless treatment you gave it.

Remember, the human back is inherently weak. Once that

weakness manifests itself, there is no reversing the tide. It is possible to surgically correct a specific back dysfunction—a so-called slipped disc, for instance—but correcting or repairing the specific problem in no way repairs the back itself.

Many great athletes have returned to their chosen careers following knee injuries, ankle injuries, shoulder injuries, torn Achilles tendons, even the most complicated leg and arm fractures. But their chances of returning to a strenuous sport after a back injury are very slight.

And it doesn't even take an injury to put someone out of action for good. It can happen just as easily via slow and gradual development.

Back pain comes in all shapes, sizes and intensities. Most people tend to think that severe and debilitating back pain—the kind that ultimately requires surgery or some other drastic corrective measure—happens only as a result of an obvious injury to the back. Therefore, unless in the beginning you suffered an injury to your back sufficiently severe to require immediate medical attention, you probably ignored the first signs of pain you had.

In a way it's unfortunate that back problems don't stem exclusively from severe injury. If they did, I would have many fewer back patients in my practice. A severe injury will usually get the victim into medical treatment right away. The problem will be diagnosed immediately and the facts of back life impressed upon the patient. The appropriate therapy will be applied and the injury, providing that it's a reparable one, as most are, will heal. Once healed, the patient will have had a thorough course on his back and will be acutely aware of the measures he or she has to take to keep the original injury from recurring and to prevent associated weaknesses from developing.

It's the more benign causes of back pain that are really the devilish ones. They are devilish because they are deceptive and lulling. Today's twinge may well be tomorrow's excruciating pain. Ninety-nine people out of a hundred would reject that assertion out of hand—until it happens to them.

Has it happened to you yet?

Whether it has or not—whether you're presently a stretcher case or still just a minor aches-and-pain sufferer—assuming your problem is one that does not need corrective surgery, *you can relieve it yourself.*

Sound unbelievable?

If you spend half your time traveling from doctor to doctor and chiropractor to chiropractor (more about that later) like Jason in search of the Golden Fleece, you may well find such a promise hard to swallow. That's understandable, because your wide-ranging peripatetic quest for relief, and hopefully a cure, indicates that you are overlooking your principal source of relief and cure—yourself.

I hate to belabor a point—but that *is* the point of this book. If you are one of the tens of millions of people in this country who suffer from common everyday backache, you can catch it before it develops into a more serious disorder. If you are one of those tens of additional millions who are already into the more serious stages of back pain, it is still not too late to reverse your condition.

With the knowledge you get from this book—about the nature of your back and the nature of its weaknesses and ailments, about what you can do to reverse the weaknesses and ailments—and with the conscientious application of that knowledge, *you need never have another backache.*

Get Off the Treatment Treadmill

If you've had back pain for any length of time you've probably jumped onto the treatment treadmill. I'm sure you might have "discovered" a particular form of treatment at one time or another that you thought was the final answer —it worked! Then, sadly, ffff! It no longer worked.

How many of you have gone the traction route? Or been subjected to adhesive strapping or braces? Long sessions with the diathermy machine? Hot and cold packs? Body casts? Chiropractic manipulation?

Some of you may already have had disc operations. Disc surgery can correct a specific disc problem, but it does not guarantee freedom from further back pain, whether associated with discs or other components of the back.

Others of you have probably gone through various forms of injection therapy.

Or perhaps simple and prolonged bed rest has been your lot.

Whichever—and there are a lot more—you've most likely found that there has been no long-term, not to mention permanent, relief. That old devil back keeps popping back into your life as surely and inevitably as spring follows winter.

The treatment treadmill is not only emotionally frustrating, it is costly. Added to the inestimable dollar loss is missed wage and salary payments due to ailing backs. The search for treatment and relief make the whole cost factor an expanding financial pyramid.

The treatment treadmill is not the answer for chronic back pain, as most of you who have been on it have learned by now. Whether you have been partial to the orthopaedist, the osteopath or the chiropractor really makes no difference. The difference is that whatever course you've pursued, it's cost you money and you've still got a weak back.

I have no desire in this book to rekindle long-standing controversies between various professional groups who take differing points of view regarding the "best" or "most effective" treatment of back problems. Any hopeful reader looking for help to free himself from the torture of his back pain isn't going to be concerned with yet another doctrinal dispute among practitioners of the healing arts. He simply wants to get his back well again and enjoy a life free from pain.

Indeed, except for informational purposes, this book is not about treatment given by others—whether by a medical doctor, osteopath, chiropractor, physical culturist, masseur, or yogi.

It's about self-therapy.

Its primary purpose is to help you get off the treatment treadmill. Although certain treatments can be helpful for certain problems of the back, the main problem of the back, as I have already intimated, lies in you.

The treatment treadmill is usually nothing but a psychological crutch most back-pain victims use to avoid facing up to the truth of their conditions. That truth is that back problems can only be licked by the people who have them.

How? Through exercise. Through specific therapeutic exercise.

The Domino Theory

Basically the human back is a framework, either flexible or rigid as circumstances dictate. From this framework every other part of the body is suspended or otherwise supported. Every part of the body is related to the back in one way or another.

The principal structure of the back—the spine—is just

about the first piece of operating machinery an embryo grows as it develops inside the womb. The spine's awesomely organized system of neurological networks directly controls every function of the body from the neck down, and a few from the neck up as well. Its beautifully precisioned bones, called vertebrae, are sturdily linked, one to the other, by some of the strongest and most durable ligaments found anywhere in the body.

This whole package is held together in suspension by associated muscles, blood vessels and bones. Except for direct injuries to or defects in the spine, most back weakness and pain start in the spine-associated structures—the muscles and the ligaments.

A strained muscle at the age of ten can just as easily lead to a ruptured intervertebral disc at thirty as can a direct traumatic blow to the same disc. Faulty posture during the growing years is just as likely to lead to acute pain in the lower back or neck at fifty as is a severe traumatic injury in an automobile accident.

The point is that most back pain in adults can be traced back to earlier weaknesses in the structure of the back that were permitted to glow like cinders in a bin of kindling until the whole bin became a raging inferno. For that's what severe and chronic back pain is—a raging inferno in your back.

As the weakness developed, usually in the musculature or in other associated structures of your back, you began to compensate for it by unconsciously holding your back in unaccustomed positions or adjusting your posture in other ways. Pretty soon, what started as a minor, localized weakness spread across and through your whole back, affecting the entire structure and, in many cases, the vertebrae and discs of the spine itself.

Had you gone to work on the small weakness at the beginning—had you allowed it the necessary time to heal and then endeavored to strengthen it—you might well have escaped your present agony.

But you didn't. And although what's past is past, the principle remains the same.

We often heard about the "domino effect" in discussions about the political and military advisability of our participation in the Vietnam War. I'm not a global strategist, so I won't presume to comment on the validity of the theory of the domino effect as it relates to America's role in the world.

I will say, however, that what you have witnessed all these months or years with respect to a breakdown of your back has been the anatomical domino effect.

Once one part of your back goes, it's not long before other parts begin to topple. Need I say more?

The only way to prevent the rest of your back from collapsing is to get in there as soon as possible and reinforce the weak link. Strengthen it! If it's too late to do that, then the next best thing is to strengthen the adjacent structures. Although the domino theory may well be obsolete politically, it is certainly not obsolete anatomically. Indeed it is more valid than ever.

Pills don't strengthen a weakened or compromised body part. Nor do injections, trusses, manipulation, diathermy, hot and cold packs, massage, or any other form of "treatment."

What strengthens any part of the anatomy compromised by injury or strain is specific exercise applied to that part after it's had a chance to heal. In the long run, it is only by strengthening weakened parts of your back—those parts that are the cause of your back pain—or strengthening adjacent parts to take up the load that the weakened part has resigned, that you will achieve *permanent* relief from your intermittent or full-time agony.

So, then, this book is dedicated to the superiority of exercise over all other forms of treatment or therapy in providing you with permanent relief from your back pain.

Not willy-nilly exercise, but a specific program of exercise designed to enable your back to take up and bear the extra loads and stresses placed on it by the earlier failure of one or more of its component parts.

There is a proper exercise regimen for every form of common back pain, be it disc-induced, muscle-induced or bone-induced. The aim of any specific regimen is to help you compensate—not through distortions of posture or through artificial devices, but through integral interior strengthening—for the weakness or weaknesses in your back that are causing you pain. Once the natural compensation is made, the pain will begin to go away. And as the rest of your back's structure increases in strength, enabling it to bear more of its gravitational and other loads, the pain will go away altogether.

These are not empty promises—I am sure you are sick to death of those by now. The application of exercise therapy works simply because it is nature's way. I've often observed in my travels around New York City what happens when an old building, sandwiched between two other buildings, is torn down. Most of the time the walls of the two adjoining buildings have to be supported with giant steel trusses to prevent them from collapsing until the cavity created by the razed building is filled up with a new structure. Had the walls of the adjoining buildings been constructed with enough structural integrity in the first place, such expensive and time-consuming shoring-up procedures could be skipped.

What you get when you get on the treatment treadmill is this same kind of artificial, expensive and time-consuming shoring up of the structures in your back. How much better, how much more sensible, to restore the integrity of the back structures themselves.

This is what you can do through exercise. The successful pursuit of such a program will not necessarily restore your back to its original structural integrity, but it will strengthen it so that at least your back pain will decrease and eventually go away altogether.

Don't think it's easy, though. Not that the exercises themselves are difficult, or painful, or terribly time-consuming. They're none of these things. In fact the exercises themselves are the easy part.

What's hard—and I've mentioned it before—is conquering your own human nature. Hopefully, after you've read through most of the book and have gotten a greater knowledge of your back and the pitfalls that await you if you neglect it any longer, you'll be ready in mind and body together to resolve to make the necessary effort. If so, you'll find in the third part of the book the specific programs that will enable you, if you pursue them diligently, to conquer your aching back.

2.

The Bones of Your Back

Man's best friends are said to be his dog and his back. This assertion may be true about the former, but if his back is man's best friend, he doesn't need enemies. Nothing has proved more unfaithful to him during his upright history than that collection of bones, ligaments, muscles and nerves known as the human back.

If you were sitting in my office now after I had just given you a general overview of your back, you would probably be bursting with questions. Your first question would most likely be, "Well, if it's all that simple, then why . . . ?"

Of course, it's not all that simple. Sure, I could easily put out a booklet of therapeutic exercises and say, "If you have this pain, do that exercise, and if you have that pain, do this one." And you might even get something out of it. But it wouldn't be enough, no matter how assiduous you were in the pursuit of the exercise program.

I've already stated that the back is an extraordinarily complicated mechanism. And it took you a long time to get to your present condition. Solving that condition is not going to be an overnight occurrence. To solve it will take not only a good deal of perseverance on the part of your will and your body, it will also demand an understanding of your back. That's what the early pages of this book are for.

So be patient. We'll get to the exercises later.

Pain and the Back

What is back pain? Definitions are necessary in order to prevent confusion. Since enough misconceptions about back pain already exist, I shall start by being simple and exact.

Back pain is any pain in the back, whether it be minor, major or catastrophic.

Ye gods, you say, that's too simple, anyone knows that. True—but, as you'll soon find out, there is pain and there is pain. Which is to say that pain in one's back may not necessarily mean that one has a back problem. Back pain can come from other sources too—it can be a symptom of ills that have no relation to the back. Back pain can indicate a diseased kidney or other organ. It can indicate a blood ailment. It can indicate a glandular problem. A tipped uterus in a woman. A swollen prostate in a man. A hernia of some kind. It can point to hip or lower joint problems. It might be a symptom of a cranial problem. There are many other organic ailments which manifest themselves, among other ways, in back pain, yet which have nothing to do with the structure or function of the back.

Now, everyone knows that the neck is connected to the backbone, that the backbone's connected to the pelvis, and the pelvis is connected to the hip bone. Not many people realize, though, that because these areas are connected they all may play a role in the production of pain.

To understand back pain and how it operates we must first gain a knowledge of the basic anatomy of the back so that we may interpret properly all the possible sources of back pain. As Abraham Lincoln once said, the best way to turn an enemy into a friend is to get to know him. I can't think of a better prescription for a bad back: get to know it!

The Basic Anatomy of Your Back

When medical students approach the study of anatomy they do so with considerable anxiety. They visualize with trepidation the vast number of new words, terms and relationships which constitute our knowledge of the structure of the body. The major reason for their fear is that they are overwhelmed by the magnitude of the material to be unerringly learned in so short a time. And they are partly right— the whole study of anatomy is pretty scary to the green student.

But having been a freshman medical student myself, having entered a medical specialty which requires an exhaustive knowledge of the human anatomy, and having taught medical students, I am better able to see the entire picture. Anatomy becomes relatively easy when one makes a broad outline and then fills in the spaces. Anatomy is logical, remarkably consistent, and has definite patterns.

Giving you a clear idea of these patterns is what I propose to do in this and the two succeeding chapters. In this way I hope to be able to describe the anatomy of the back and its related structures so that you will not only have a clear picture of the architecture of the back but will also absorb this knowledge in sufficient detail to enable you to properly understand and deal with your own back pain. Who knows, you may even want to continue the study and go on to master Gray's *Anatomy*.

The Spine

Next to the human brain, man's spine has been the most significant factor in his evolution—not only for the ills it has caused him, but because it is the one component of man's structural make-up that enabled him, millions of years ago, to stand erect. It freed his hands from the need to support him, at rest or in motion. As a result of his arms and hands being freed to operate independently of his legs and feet, and with the aid of his brain, man has gained dominion over all the earth.

Both man's hands and his brain depend upon his spine. It is no exaggeration to say that your backbone is the backbone of all human achievement.

By the same token, your personal backbone, the one that gets the aches and pains you are now seeking to overcome, is as much as any other the one part of the body that can make you or break you. Curiously, to most people it is also one of the least familiar parts, notwithstanding the fact that it is the part that most people see the least of. Perhaps it's simply a case of out of sight, out of mind.

But whether you see it or you don't, one thing is certain. Your spine and the structures surrounding it go to make up one truly amazing hunk of machinery.

Your spine serves three purposes:

1. It is a support structure for your body, anchoring the ribs and connecting your head with your pelvis.

2. It is a housing unit for your spinal cord, which controls your body's nervous system.

3. It is the primary instrument of your body's flexibility, by virtue of its unique construction.

Let's look at an illustration of the spine or backbone and see what its structure is all about and what makes it so important and unique in your life. Figure 1 is a diagrammatic representation of the spine.

For purposes of illustration we can divide the spine into four regions. These regions are identified by the specific characteristics of their vertebrae (the bones of the spinal column). We find:

1. *The Cervical Spine, or the Neck Region.* This region consists of seven vertebral bones, or vertebrae. Vertebrae are small bony structures that make up the backbone (more on these a little further on). The main characteristics of the seven cervical vertebrae are their extraordinary range of motion. In addition to supporting the head, their mobility permits the head to move through its wide spectrum.

2. *The Thoracic or Dorsal Spine, or Mid-Back Region.* Twelve vertebrae form this area. Special connections are present for the attachment of the ribs. Because of the attachment of the ribs, this area of the spine is relatively immobile.

3. *The Lumbar Spine, or Lower Back Region.* The brunt of the weight of the upper body is borne by the five large vertebrae here. They are broader and heavier than the ones above in order to support the large mass of the upper body. In addition, very large muscles attach to these vertebrae. This is the area in which the ever-popular ailment known as lumbago resides.

4. *The Sacrum and Coccyx Region.* The sacrum constitutes the base of the spine. It is a broad, triangular structure attached at the top to the lumbar region of the spine and on the sides to the pelvis. In the development of the embryo in a mother's womb, five separate bones are formed. They eventually fuse and form a single bone structure—the *sacrum.* The *coccyx* (pronounced "cox-ix") is the collection of a few small bones which come off the end of the sacrum. It is probably the remnant of what was once man's tail in his early anthropological period.

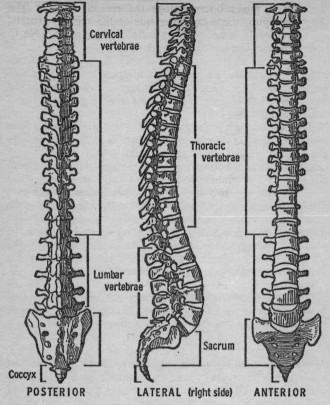

FIG. 1   Three-part view of the spine.

This, then, is the basic frame of your spine or backbone. All in all, your spinal column is composed of twenty-four oddly shaped but generally flat bits of bone (the vertebrae) sitting one on top of the other from your neck to the base of your spine.

If you were able to remove one of your lumbar vertebrae from your back for a moment and lay it flat on a table, it would appear generally circular, with three bone spurs or projections extending from the rear portion, as in Figures 2 and 3. If you reach back and press your finger against your backbone you will be able to feel the center projection, which is called in medical terminology the *spinous process*. The other two spurs, those on either side of the spinous process, are more deeply imbedded in muscle and you're not able to feel them from outside.

The middle projection bends slightly downward, overlapping the vertebra below, so that all together these twenty-four center spurs serve to protect your spinal cord in much the same way that the overlapping shingles on the roof of a house keep the rain out.

The two side projections, each of which are known as the *transverse process*, provide anchorage for the muscles you use for twisting and bending your back.

On the top and bottom surfaces, between the spinous process and the two transverse processes, there are four vertical bone projections, two on top and two below, which are roughly half an inch in diameter. These are known as *articular facets* and they fit against equivalent projections on the vertebrae immediately above and below to act as joints. I'll be mentioning these more than once because not only are they important connections between the vertebrae, they're occasionally the villains in a number of backache plots.

But that's not all there is to a vertebra. There is also the body of the vertebra, a thick, flat, semi-circular bone that makes up the front part of the vertebra. This is the main weight-bearing platform of each of the vertebrae, although it shares the load with the articular facets.

Running right through the vertebra from top to bottom, between the spinous process in the rear and the body of the vertebra in front, is a hole. This hole, aligned with the corresponding holes in each of the other vertebrae in your spine, comprise a continuous tunnel called the spinal canal. This canal contains the spinal cord. The hole itself is called the *vertebral foramen*.

Now take a look at a partial view of the spine with the vertebrae assembled for business. You will see in Figure 4 that each vertebral body is joined to the next by a capsule of layered ligament and other tissue that is roughly flat and circular in shape. These capsules encase, like jelly within a doughnut, a gelatinous substance known as the *nucleus pulposis*. The more popular name for this entire affair is "disc," as in "slipped disc."

A pair of tough cartilaginous plates, again flat and circular in shape, form the top and bottom of the capsule. Be-

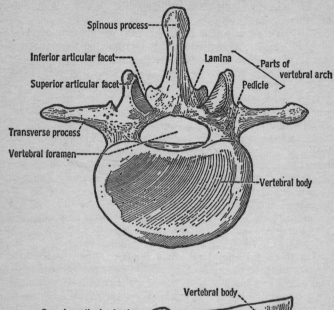

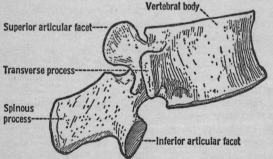

FIGS. 2 & 3   View of a lumbar vertebra from two angles, noting all parts.

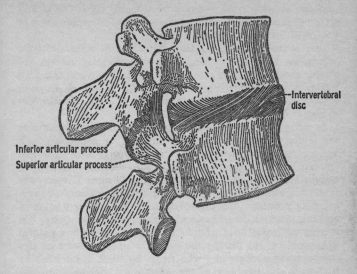

Intervertebral disc

Inferior articular process

Superior articular process

FIG. 4   A sideview of the lumbar region of the spine, showing the relationship of vertebrae and discs.

tween these plates and the encircling tissue is the disc itself, the nucleus pulposis.

These discs and the twenty-four vertebrae make up the spine or backbone. If any of them are damaged, injured, diseased or otherwise thrown out of whack, you're going to hurt, but good.

If the spine was without discs and the vertebrae were required to grind against each other, your back would not last long. The function of the discs is to separate the vertebrae and prevent them from rubbing against one another. The discs act like an hydraulic system, their jelly-like interiors dispersing pressure evenly in all directions along your back.

The importance of discs and their function are obvious when you consider the tremendous loads placed upon the spine by gravity alone, and the additional stresses caused by bending, walking, running, jumping and lifting. Alf Nachemson of Sweden, a celebrated orthopaedic surgeon who has done a considerable amount of research on the back, calculated that when an able-bodied man bends over to pick up a

fifty-pound weight, he exerts a pressure of six hundred and
sixty pounds at the juncture of the lumbar and sacral spine in
the lower back.

Our intervertebral discs are constructed to withstand such
forces. As long as they and their supporting structures are
strong and healthy, the discs can survive. It is when the discs
begin to weaken, whether through age, injury or through
neglect of less serious back problems, that trouble develops.

In early life—childhood and adolescence—the disc spaces
are wide, the disc substance a true gel or semi-fluid, and
the hydraulic system very efficient. However, with age—and
by age I mean from twenty-five years onward—changes in
the disc structure of your back begin to occur. They slowly
lose their semi-gel quality, scarring begins, desiccation (dry-
ing out) proceeds, and the spaces narrow. These are signs of
natural, gradual deterioration. It happens to everybody, but
it does not mean that everybody will end up with a painful
disc problem. It's usually the person who is unaware of this
deterioration process and who treats his back in later life as
if it were still the back of his youth on whom disc troubles
descend.

An active eighty-year-old can have fairly good discs,
whereas a sedentary thirty-year-old may have horrible ones.
Why the difference? What determines the continuation of
healthy discs or the rapid deterioration of others?

Certainly hereditary factors play a role in the fate of
the nucleus pulposes. But I feel very strongly, along with most
orthopaedic and neurosurgeons, that abnormal stresses, poor
or neglected musculature and sudden injuries play an even
more dramatic part in producing extrusion or protrusion of
an intervertebral disc or in accelerating its deterioration.
(I shall discuss these problems at greater length and in more
detail when we reach the chapter on the slipped disc.)

The Pelvis

The spine is not all there is to the bone structure of the
back. At its bottom end the backbone rests on a tricky
combination of three more bones, which I'm sure everybody
has heard of or talked about at one time or another.

One is called the sacrum, and the other two, flanking it,
are the *ilia*. Where the ilia bones are attached by ligaments to

either side of the triangular sacrum, the famous "sacroilac" joint is found.

The two ilia are joined to the sides of the sacrum and are connected in front by a strong, dense ligament known as the *symphysis pubis*. This arrangement is what we know as the pelvis.

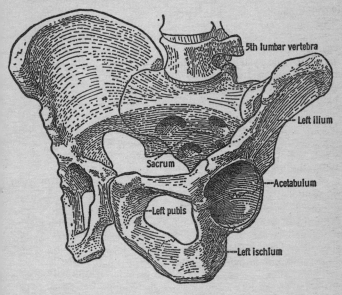

FIG. 5 A frontal view of the pelvic area, with the backbone descending to the pelvis, and all the anatomical (skeletal) features of the pelvic area noted.

The pelvis is the floor on which the lower internal organs rest, such as the bladder, the rectum, the large intestine and, in the female, the uterus. Because of its configuration and its attachments, the pelvis is relatively immobile. No motion whatsoever is present at the front of the pelvis, and only a small amount of mobility occurs at the sacroiliac joint.

On either side of the pelvis are two sockets, the *acetabula*, into which the ball-like ends of the thigh bones fit. These sockets are the hip joints. The motion provided by these ball-and-socket joints is great indeed, allowing you to walk, run, climb stairs, stoop, squat, sit, straddle a chair, ride a horse, kick a ball, even to ski and swim.

Your pelvis, then, is the connecting structure between your spine and your lower extremities—your hips and legs. It provides support and stability, but has little mobility itself. The pelvis of the male and the female have different shapes because of the child-bearing function in the female, but otherwise there are no sexual differences.

In many cases the lower spine and the sacroiliac joint are the main actors in the tragic drama of an aching back. But there's another bit player that manages to sneak on stage once in a while and steal the show. That's the coccyx, and this little pest is worth a brief look.

Like the sacrum, the coccyx is composed of three or four (depending on the individual) bones which fuse together. About two inches long, it attaches to the lower point of the sacrum with a slightly movable joint. It provides an anchorage for some of the small muscles in your rectal area that are essential to the control of bowel movement.

The tail-like configuration of the coccyx lends credence to the notion that the coccyx is what's left of the tail we might have had before we came down out of the trees. It seldom gives much trouble and is usually not associated with the kind of back pain we're concerned about here. However, if you've ever sat down on a chair that wasn't there or have slipped on an icy sidewalk and landed flush on the base of your spine, you know the kind of pain it's capable of.

There, then, are the key items in the skeletal or bone structure of the back. Connecting the skeleton in this simple way has certainly not been a difficult task. So far I have shown you the bones and the skeletal regions of your back, described the structures and functions and noted their relationship to one another.

The twenty-four vertebrae, with a disc cushion between each, constitute the spine. Joined with the bone structures on which the spine rests—the sacroiliac and the pelvis—the two comprise the basic foundation of your back.

But what would a foundation be without a house on top of it?

3.

The Ligaments and Muscles of Your Back

Man is more than bones. If we continue the analogy of the spine being like the foundation of a house, we know that a foundation must be cemented together to be an effective supporting base.

In the case of your spine, the mortar that holds the dry foundation bricks—the bones—together are your ligaments, cartilages, tendons and muscles. The entire package amounts to a mechanism that can bend and twist, turn and squirm, shake and wriggle, and do just about anything else within the range of human motion—as long as it remains healthy. Just as easily, it can stiffen up, hold itself rigid in just about any position, and can exert peak power whenever we need it— again, as long as it remains healthy.

The Ligaments

Any sports fan knows the importance of ligaments. "Joe Namath has torn ligaments in both knees and cannot run." "Claude Killy almost tore the ligaments in his right ankle during the slalom." "Bill Russell tore some ligaments in his back and missed ten games." Indeed, ligaments are important. They're the things that hold our spines, as well as other parts of our bodies, together. But what are they, really? What are they made of, how do they work, and what happens when they get torn?

Ligaments are thick, dense, very tough strands of tissue which *attach one bone to another*. Do not confuse them with tendons, which are similar in structure but different in function—tendons *attach muscles to bones*.

Ligaments go from bone to bone and hold them together in their proper relationships. They are flexible, in order for motion to occur, but at the same time they have a low degree of elasticity. Thus, they can be stretched only a limited amount before they tear or rupture.

Once a ligament has been completely torn, it does not repair itself. It can only be repaired surgically, that is, through the procedure of removing the section of ligament that is torn, then employing other tissue to replace it. If a torn or ruptured ligament is not repaired, its check-rein effect is lost and abnormal motion can occur at the involved joint. This instability can lead to actual damage of the joint surfaces and of other supporting structures. If left uncorrected, pain and loss of function result.

Numerous ligaments connect and hold the foundation blocks of the spine—the vertebrae, the sacrum and the pelvis—together. A few of these deserve a closer look because of the disability and pain they can produce if they are damaged. Figure 6 gives a clear picture of the major ligament components of the back and how they function.

1. *Interspinous Ligaments*. These are the bands that travel from one spinous process to another over the entire length of the spine. They relax with extension of the spine (bending backward) but become tight with flexion (bending forward), and thus help to limit the motion which can occur between each of the vertebrae. Occasionally, when sudden severe flexion of the spine occurs, these ligaments may tear or rupture and cause localized pain for long periods of time.

2. *Intertransverse Ligaments*. These extend between the transverse process on either side of the vertebra and hold the vertebrae together along these two axes. They are best developed in the lumbar region of the spine and help to keep you from bending too far to one side or the other.

3. *The Ligamentum Flavum*. This is a dense, yellow-hued ligament which binds the rear segments of the vertebrae and forms the roof of the spinal canal. This ligament

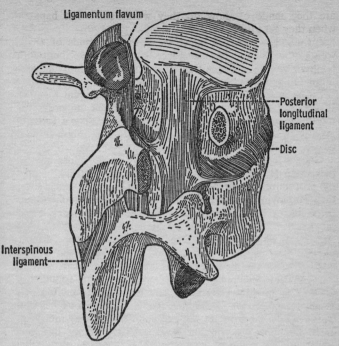

Ligamentum flavum

Posterior longitudinal ligament

Disc

Interspinous ligament

FIG. 6   A rear view of two vertebrae with ligaments.

acts as a protective covering for the spinal cord and the nerve roots and is more elastic than the other ligaments.

4. *The Annulus Fibrosus.* This ligament connects each vertebra to the next in a circumferential manner and contains the nucleus pulposis, popularly called the disc. The annulus fibrosus is an extremely strong ligament composed of multiple layers. Each layer is in a radial relationship to the others in order to increase its strength. The tire industry has copied this arrangement of nature and the result is the radial ply tire. Although the annulus fibrosus also serves to restrict excessive motion between the vertebrae, its most important function is to hold the vertebral disc in place and contain the disc for the cushion effect.

5. *The Anterior and Posterior Longitudinal Ligaments.* These two long ligaments extend from the top of the

spine to the sacrum at the bottom, one in front and one in back of the bodies of the vertebrae. As these ligaments cross the spaces between the vertebrae they blend with the annulus fibrosus and reinforce it. The front ligament of this pair, the one that runs along the stomach-side of your spine, is much thicker and stronger than the rear one, which separates the bodies from the spinal canal.

All these ligaments are elastic to a certain degree and provide the spine with mobility.

The Muscles

Muscle is composed of contractible fibers which are responsive to nervous impulses. The actual physiology of the nerve structures and muscle reaction is quite complicated. It is sufficient for our purposes to know that all skeletal muscles (those muscles which are attached to the bones and are responsible for the motion of our skeletons) are controlled by our conscious thought processes.

This is in contrast to our intetnal organs, such as the heart, stomach and intestines, which have muscles within them but whose muscles are not controlled by voluntary impulse or conscious thought. You can not simply will your heart to slow down or your stomach to stop growling when you're hungry. But you certainly can will yourself to pick up a ball, run a little faster or slower, or scratch your ear.

All muscles have nerves which originate in the brain, descend through the spinal cord and branch out into the muscles. One nerve may supply branches to many muscles. Or one muscle may have several branches from different nerves. Therefore the contraction of a muscle may be either partial or complete, depending upon the activity of the nerves which supply it. This activity in turn depends upon the control of the brain.

I will get into the nervous system and the role it plays in the anatomy of the back in more detail in the next chapter. For now let us consider your nerves as a two-way street. They carry impulses from your brain to your muscles and from the muscles to the brain.

Those portions of your nerves which travel from your brain to your muscles are called the *efferent* fibers. Those portions which carry the nature of your muscular response back to your brain and confirm your mental command are called the *afferent* fibers. Your nerves are capable not only of initiating contraction of your muscles but, because of their instantaneous feed-back system, the rapidity, intensity and relaxation of your muscles can be controlled. Not a bad computer system, eh?

The muscles associated with your back operate like all your other muscles. A brain cell is activated which sends impulses along specific nerves that run through your spinal cord and branch out into your musculature. These impulses instantaneously stimulate a muscle or a group of muscles and cause them to contract.

The specific muscles we are interested in here are those which are associated with and support your spine—what are generally known as the back muscles.

Do not be fooled by the phrase "back muscles" though. When we talk of back muscles we do not mean just the muscles *in* your back. We mean both the muscles *in* and the muscles *associated with* your back. As you'll see, muscles that are not actually in your back can play a very significant role in the production of back pain.

There are four general muscle groups that affect your back. They are:

1. *The abdominal muscles,* which provide frontal support for the back by keeping your stomach and other anterior areas of your body in line.

2. *The extensor muscles* of the spine, which provide posterior support by holding the rear frame of your torso erect.

3. *The lateral muscles,* which provide lateral support and motion.

4. *The hip muscles,* which, by virtue of their relationship to the pelvis, affect the spine.

Although I have listed these four muscle groups separately, it is important that you understand that they are thoroughly synergistic—they work together, are interdependent, and are all essential to the proper function of your back—especially the first three.

If you were to attempt to hold a long pole vertically erect with three guy wires, each wire would have to exert a pull equal to the other two. If one wire is weak, or slack, regardless of how strong the other two are, the pole will not re-main vertical. It will sag in the direction of the other two wires, an abnormal motion.

Your spine acts similarly. The three muscle groups are equivalent to the three wires. If one group is weak, either due to paralysis or to lack of exercise, abnormal motion of the spine occurs and damage results.

The Abdominal Muscles

These muscles support your abdominal wall. They extend from the rib cage to the sides and to the front of the pelvis, and are attached to these structures by tendons—strong, tough tissues similar to ligaments.

The abdominal muscles are composed of distinct sub-groups which are identified as follows:

1. the *rectus abdominus*
2. the *internal oblique*
3. the *external oblique*
4. the *transverse abdominus*

Although I separate these muscle sub-groups for the purpose of explanation, since they act together we can consider them as a unit. These muscles, in addition to supporting the con-tents of your abdominal cavity, help to control the bending movements of your spine. And when they are tensed, they help to relieve strain on your back. Let's consider them as your anterior guy wires.

The Extensor Muscles

These muscles, which lie along the spine itself, are also known as the *spine extensors*. They consist of many layers of muscle with complicated names which we need not go into here. Some of the muscles are very small and span short dis-tances, in certain cases only an inch. Others are vast and ex-tend from your neck to your sacrum, which, you'll remem-ber, is at the bottom of your spine. Generally the larger muscles lie close to the skin, while the smaller ones are nearer the bones. But they all act in harmony, whether just a small segment or the entire mass. They attach to the spine, the pelvis, the ribs and the head through the medium of connecting tendons. These muscles get their heaviest play when you arch your back, hold your spine stiff and erect, and push or pull some heavy weight.

The Lateral Muscles

The lateral, or side, muscles are pretty well hidden. These lie against the side walls of your spine. Two major subgroups in this set are the most active performers here:

1. the *quadratus lumborum*
2. the *psoas major*

The quadratus lumborum muscles help control the side bending of your spine. They come into play in such activities as dancing and gymnastics. I remember this muscle group well, for as a medical student I was told that it was responsible for a woman's wiggle when she walks. How many people would have guessed that Marilyn Monroe owed at least part of her success to her quadratus lumborum?

The psoas major muscle is one of the largest single muscles in your body. It is present on both sides of your spine—it passes from the spine through the pelvis and attaches to the top of the thigh bone just below the hip joint. Thus the psoas major affects not only your back, but your hips as well. It is called a "two-joint" muscle because it acts on more than one joint.

These three muscle groups—the abdominals, extensors and laterals—constitute the basic supporting structure of your back. However, as I have indicated, your hips can not be divorced from your back because of their intrinsic relationship to your pelvis.

What, you might ask, do the hips have to do with problems in the back? The answer will soon be clear.

Each of your hips has four groups of muscles which support it and contribute to its mobility. By virtue of the relationship of the hip to the pelvis, and that of the pelvis to the spine, what goes on in the hip can have a very significant effect on the back. This is mainly due to the four muscle groups of the hip. They are:

1. the *hip flexors*
2. the *hip abductors*
3. the *hip adductors*
4. the *hip extensors*

The hip flexors lie along the front of your hip and act in such a way as to enable you to bring your thigh upwards. This muscle group consists of the *sartorius, rectus femoris, ilial psoas,* and portions of the *tensor fascia lata* muscles.

The hip abductors lie along the side of your hip and extend from the top of the pelvis to the *greater trochanter* of the thigh bone. The abductors are made up of the *gluteus medius* and *gluteus minimus* muscles, both of which provide stability for the hip and allow you to engage in such activities as standing on one foot.

The hip adductors (notice the difference between "ab" and "ad") are your groin muscles, which enable you to pull your legs together and also provide stability in the pelvic region. This muscle group is made up of the *adductor brevis, longus* and *magnus* muscles, as well as the *pectineus* and *gracilis* muscles. This gracefully named muscle, because it holds the legs together, has often been referred to as the guardian of virginity. At least in days of yore!

Finally, the hip extensors are the massive muscles which lie along the back of your hip joint. The most prominent muscle in this group is the *gluteus maximus,* known among body builders and weight lifters as the "glutes." They form the major portion of your derriere and are what you flex when you tuck in your buttocks. This muscle has a practical function as well—as it passes behind your hip it becomes the main muscle you use when you climb stairs. Running power and speed come from this muscle too. Additional hip extensors are the hamstring muscles, which are two-joint muscles. They extend from the pelvis down the back of the thigh and insert below the knee into the lower leg bones. They are used primarily for extending the hip and are also responsible for the flexing of your knee.

The hip extensor muscles as a group control *lumbar lordosis,* which, when excessive, produces "swayback," a condition painfully prevalent in many people. These muscles, combined with the hip flexors, are extremely important in maintaining good posture—something I'll get to in a later chapter.

There, then, you have a glimpse of the second major component of your back's structure. Taken together—your back-bone, the ligaments that glue it all together, and the muscles and tendons that support it—it is quite a remarkable mechanism. Given proper care, a fair shake, and a little understanding, your back will take on any job you ask of it, including its primary job of carrying you around on your feet.

When it fails, in practically all of the most severe cases the failure arises out of some weakness in one or more of the various components. Such an unhappy condition is generally called instability, and when instability occurs the odds are good that it will launch a virulent case of lumbago, sciatica or the general miseries.

Remember my example of the three guy wires? Unless there is a basic defect in the spine, weakness and pain usually develop because the spine is not being held in its proper position for prolonged periods of time. Like the pole that leans away from the vertical because one of its supporting wires has become slack, your spine will do the same thing when one of the three main muscle groups that supports it weakens. And therein lies the story of most common back pain.

Not that the spine is supposed to be straight, mind you. It's not. Unlike Nelson's Column in London's Trafalgar Square, the spinal column is not a perpendicular structure with one stone or bone balanced directly on top of the one below it. Partly for strength and mobility, and partly to accommodate the organs of the body, but mainly because that's the way it happened, the spinal column is a curved structure.

Man's spine must be supple and stable. It must be capable of being balanced upright or held rigid in many other positions. Although it must be strong, it must allow free movement in many directions. To provide stability and flexibility, strength and free movement—all these things at once—is quite an engineering problem. The answer to this problem has been evolved with superb design and ingenuity through the more than a million years since man first adopted the upright posture. The solution has not produced any cumbersome reinforcing bands of supporting structures. It has all been achieved with grace and beauty.

That's why it is so painful, figuratively, to see it abused. Yet abuse it we do—every day of our lives. And when we do it often enough, the pain we experience is no longer figurative. It is real.

Pain is associated with the nervous system. It is the nerves that let us know we are having pain. In the next chapter we'll get closer to the whole concept of pain—back pain in general and your pain specifically. We shall explore together just how and why back pain manifests itself.

4.

The Nerves
of Your Back

"Wow, what nerve he has!" Or, "Hey, that really took some nerve." How many times in your life have you heard such statements?

To say someone has nerve is almost the direct opposite of calling someone spineless or without backbone. Nerve is one of those qualities we admire in other people and in ourselves. Perhaps that's because nerves are associated in our minds with pain, and when someone does something that "takes a lot of nerve" we know that he is exposing himself to a good deal of pain if what he is attempting to do doesn't succeed.

Did you ever notice, by the way, how often many of the metaphors we use for the purposes of praise or condemnation relate to the back? I would guess that next to sexual metaphors, the use of back-related metaphors is most frequent in our language. An indication, perhaps, that next to sex the back is our most frequent source of concern.

The Nature of Back Pain

Pain is the great leveler of all men. It respects no one. Whether you are a private or a general, a truck driver or the Chairman of General Motors, a so-called bookworm or a hard-nosed football player, a contented housewife or a women's liberationist, a homosexual or a heterosexual, a man or a woman—one thing you all share in common is pain. And a nervous system.

We are all aware of pain. It's true that some people have

a greater tolerance for pain than others, but the ability to withstand it has nothing to do with the nervous system itself. This greater tolerance or higher threshold of pain that some people have over others is due to psychological factors and to a certain degree of pre-conditioning.

What I am pointing out is that we all have the same basic nervous system, and no matter the degree of our psychological ability to withstand pain, we all have a breaking point. This is the point where pain is no longer something we can withstand or resist.

When fear or unaccustomed stimuli occur, pain may be enhanced and intensified. How often do you turn your head away when a doctor is about to give you an injection? You do this in anticipation of pain, and usually are quite surprised to learn afterwards that you hardly felt the needle go in.

The boxer in the ring can take several severe blows to the head and body without feeling much pain. But if you or I get socked in the face it hurts. This is because the boxer is pre-conditioned to take the blows, whereas we are not.

So we all experience pain. Our reactions to it can be greater or lesser, depending on what fears we have in association with it or what pre-conditioning we've had with respect to it. But the plain fact remains that no matter what our reactions are, pain is unpleasant.

Wouldn't it be nice if we never had pain at all? Imagine no pain. Needles would not hurt, cuts and bruises would go unnoticed, babies would be born without any discomfort to their mothers, everyone would go to the dentist with a smile on his face. Indeed, no one would ever have back pain and I would not be writing this book.

Such a utopian state would be a dangerous one. *Pain is necessary*. It's as necessary to us as seeing, eating, hearing and procreating. The human race could not survive without pain.

Pain is a fascinating subject. Oh, I agree, it's certainly not very fascinating to someone who's experiencing it. The only fascination there lies in finding relief. Nevertheless, as an objective study, pain *is* fascinating because it tells us so much —not only about disease and injury, but about human nature itself.

Back pain is like all other pain. It hurts, sometimes excruciatingly so. But it's different too. The difference lies in the fact that back pain so often causes disability, whether short-term or long-term, whether occasional or frequent.

You can have a severe toothache and still get through your day, however uncomfortably. You can have a headache, a stomach ache, a charley horse, an ingrown toenail—any number of painful conditions—and still manage to function. All of these can be relieved in fairly short and simple order and, once relieved, will stay away.

Not always so with back pain. An attack of acute back pain will knock you for a loop, and unlike most other kinds of pain it will keep coming back to haunt you. A dentist can repair your defective tooth in no time and relieve the pain permanently. A doctor can not repair your defective back in "no time." True, he might be able to relieve the pain—temporarily—but your back, as we have already seen, is a much more complicated item than a tooth.

The great majority of my back patients ended up in my office to begin with because they were the kind of optimists who just did not realize that when their backs first started to act up they were in for something serious. They shrugged off their initial bouts of back pain on the theory that, since the pain came by itself, it would obligingly depart the same way.

Now I'm all in favor of optimists. There's nothing that cheers me more than to have one of my patients breeze into my office with a merry "Hi, Doctor, it's getting better!" These patients have good reason for optimism, for they are the ones who have embarked on a program at home to rebuild their backs.

It's the false optimists who concern me. And anyone who believes his back pain is going to go away of its own accord, or who believes that the pharmaceutical relief of his pain is going to cure his back, or even that manipulative, medical or surgical corrective measures are going to entirely solve the problems created by his back, is a false optimist.

The Back and the Nervous System

In order to understand your back pain, you should first understand your nervous system. I'm sure all of you know that pain is a function of the nervous system, but I'm constantly amazed at how little those of you who experience chronic back pain understand about how and why this relationship exists. Perhaps a better understanding of your nervous system and how it relates to your back would help you to deal with your pain in a more effective way.

It has become fashionable these days to compare the brain to a computer, as if that makes it easier for us to understand what the brain is. Perhaps it does make it easier —for the computer expert. But I'm not a computer expert. Nor, I dare say, are most of you.

Basically your brain is the master control system of the entire organism that is your body. What it controls is a vast network of what we call nerves—of varying size and of great quantity—which in turn control and effect every single portion of your body.

A nerve is a cordlike or filamentous band of tissue made up essentially of fibers. Thousands of these, large and small, are to be found in the body, the major ones radiating from centers in the brain through the spinal cord to all parts of the body. The incredibly complex network of nerves throughout the body is known as the nervous system.

The nervous system, then, comprises the nerve cells which exist in the gray matter of the brain and which are collectively dispersed throughout the body in the form of fibrous cords or strands of fibrous tissue of all lengths and thicknesses. The system coordinates and regulates the excitation of muscles, organs and glands and directly conditions all behavior and consciousness.

In vertebrates, including man, the nervous system has two major parts—the *somatic* system and the *autonomic* system. The somatic system is the combination of brain and spinal-cord nerves which govern our voluntary actions, motions and sensory feelings. The autonomic system is part of the peripheral system that governs our involuntary actions, motions and feelings, such as those having to do with our vascular and nutritive functions, i.e., heartbeat and digestion. Both systems are interrelated and are components of our central nervous system, but for our purposes here we are more concerned with the somatic system.

Some nerves—receptors—are mainly "sensory." That is, they receive stimuli from the world about us and instantaneously transmit the sensations received back to the brain center, where the information is interpreted and acted upon.

A simple example of this is when you accidentally place your finger on a hot stove. The nerve endings in your finger are immediately stimulated (your nerves have special hot and cold sensory endings, as well as endings for other sensations) and an electrical charge is flashed through your nervous system to the brain. The brain receives this informational impulse and refers it to an "action center." The action center sends an impulse down along an effector or "motor" nerve—a nerve that controls the muscles associated with the finger and its nerve endings—and suddenly the finger is abruptly withdrawn from the stove. The entire sequence occurs a hundred times faster than the blink of an eye. We all have actually experienced it, or something like it, thousands of times in our lives.

The same process holds true for sharp objects, broken bones, and innumerable other pain-inducing stimuli. Imagine walking on a broken leg and not knowing that it was broken. Within a short time the leg would be destroyed. If we carry this logic to its conclusion it becomes obvious that pain serves a very good purpose. It is our primary warning system. It informs us when anything is wrong.

Now, the back is not only important as the supporting structure of the rest of our bodies, it also serves another purpose. Like the skull which protects the brain, the spine provides continuous protection to that vital part of our nervous system which allows the whole process of sensation and pain to happen in the first place. Thus in addition to our brain and our nerves, for our nervous system to work we need the transmission system—the spinal cord.

The brain is the storehouse of our knowledge, the seat of our memory, the factory of our thought, and the origin of our will. As a result of our mental processes, the brain decides to move or not to move a part of our body. A message has to be sent from the specific brain cell to corresponding muscles at distant parts of the body which carry out its command. The message is sent out through a nerve fiber. Thousands of these nerve fibers are collected together in a vital trunk line of communication between the brain and the outlying parts of the body. This trunk line is the spinal cord.

The spinal cord also contains nerve fibers which travel in the opposite direction, for messages from outlying parts of the body have to be carried back to the brain. The brain must be kept fully informed at all times of what is going on at the periphery.

At every level in the spinal cord there are groups of nerve cells that receive messages via the sensory nerves, and other groups of cells which send off messages about such things as motion via the motor nerves. This is how the whole "hot-stove" process, and its thousands of possible equivalents, work.

A motor nerve root emerges from each side of the spinal cord at the level of each vertebra along the spine, where it separates into several branches which "mix" with branches of other nerve roots and spread through the body. For each motor root going from the brain and spinal cord into the body in this fashion, a sensory root returns from the body and joins the back of the spinal cord.

Altogether there are thirty pairs of mixed spinal nerves, and they enter or leave the spinal cord through small holes in the vertebrae known as *foramens*.

In the case of the brain, protection of this most vital nerve center of the body is provided by the fact that it's encased in a rigid, strong box of bone—the skull. It is not possible to protect the spinal cord this way because, as we have seen, movement has to be permitted throughout the spine.

Protection and movement, however, are both allowed for in the construction of the spine by its having a hole running through all the vertebrae. When all the holes of the vertebrae are lined up they form a tunnel of bone known as the spinal canal. This canal provides strong protection to the spinal cord but at the same time permits considerable movement of the spine.

One interesting anatomical point should be brought out now. The spinal cord only occupies the upper two-thirds of the spinal canal. It terminates at the level of the first lumbar vertebra. Although in the infant the spinal cord extends the entire length of the spinal canal from the skull to the sacrum, the growth of the cord does not keep up with the longitudinal growth of the spine itself. By the time we reach adulthood, then, our spinal cord only reaches as far as the first lumbar vertebra, just below the area where the last rib is attached. However the nerves, or the lumbar nerve roots as they are called at this point, extend downward and continue to emerge on either side of the lower vertebrae and the sacrum in a regular and symmetrical manner.

So in spite of the fact that the spinal cord does not traverse the entire spine, the lumbar nerve roots travel downward inside the spinal canal from the end of the cord and emerge from their correct spaces between the last five vertebrae. It will be seen later that the presence of these lumbar nerves inside the lumbar spinal canal is an important factor

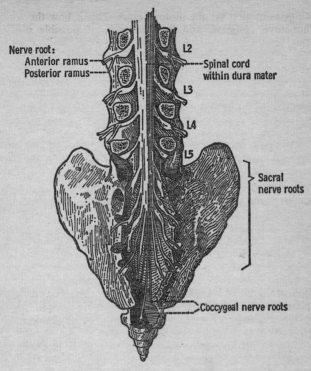

Nerve root:
Anterior ramus
Posterior ramus

L2
L3
L4
L5

Spinal cord
within dura mater

Sacral
nerve roots

Coccygeal nerve roots

*FIG. 7 Detail of spinal cord running through
spine, with nerve—motor and sensory—branches,
plus mixed spinal nerves.*

in the production of pain and other symptoms of the slipped
disc.

Now we have a concept of the nervous system, with its
central cells located either in the brain or in the spinal cord
and with branches that go to all our muscles, blood vessels,
ligaments, bones, internal and external organs, even to the
skin. Some of the branches are receptors of sensory stimuli,
or *afferent* nerves—they take a reaction back to the main
cell in our brain via the spinal cord. Other branches are ef-
fectors, or *efferent* nerves—they carry the brain's reaction
and exert a motor effect upon a specific area of the body.

Man has the most complex brain and nervous system ever developed. The computer is really only a pale imitation.

All the nerve cells and their branches have interconnecting links so that very few isolated activities occur. Specialized central cells exist for specific activities, and they have their own special branches. But like the muscle groups discussed in the last chapter, our nervous systems are a completely integrated network with each part of the system playing a role in the workings of the whole.

We see, then, that the nervous system plays a very important part in the general anatomy of the back. The spine serves not only to *protect* a vital portion of the nervous system, it also acts as the final common pathway of neural energy between the brain and the rest of the body.

But what about specific back pain? What does this have to do with the nervous system?

Back Pain and the Nervous System

I have already mentioned the painful aspects of sensation as brought to us through the sensory nerves. Let me say as an aside that although we owe the pain we endure to these nerves, to them we also owe the sensations of pleasure we enjoy. Just as, through them, we feel the burn of a flame or the sear of an inflamed tooth, we are also able to perceive a spectrum of beautiful colors, taste delicious foods, hear melodious songs and experience the pleasurable warmth of a loved one's caresses.

Your back is part of nature and it exists in a balance of all sorts of opposing forces. When your back is in a normal state of health, you experience neither pain nor pleasure from it. When everything is working properly—when all your vertebral bones are well-aligned and properly spaced, when your spinal ligaments and back-associated muscles and tendons are in their proper tensions, and when your spinal cord is functioning without interference—there is no reason why you *should* have pleasurable sensations in your back, or painful ones. The only pleasure you might receive is a spiritual one, the kind that derives from your sense of security about your back.

But let something go wrong, let the balance get tipped, and pain is your reward. Not only the spiritual pain that comes from worry or anxiety about the state of your health, but real live pain—the kind that hurts a specific part of your body.

Back pain comes in a variety of shapes, sizes and intensities. These all depend on a number of things—the nature of a disorder, the site in your back where the disorder occurs, and the cause. Notwithstanding all of these, though, the real source of the pain you feel in your back, whether mild or excruciating, is your sensory nerves. Note that I said they are the source, not the cause, of your pain.

Your nervous system operates on your back in just the same way it operates on the rest of your body. Remember the "hot-stove" example I used before? Well, your back is full of hot-stove possibilities too.

Your back is one vast and complex system of nerves hooked into your main nervous system. You've got big nerves, medium-sized nerves, small nerves, tiny nerves, miniscule nerves, thousands of them, all running to various points in your back. Every last and least part in your back is attached to your nervous system, and vice versa.

When you burn your finger on a hot stove, the cluster of sensory nerve endings in your finger flash the message through the incredibly complex circuit of your nervous system to your brain, which in turn flashes back the command through your finger's effector nerve circuit that enables you to lift your finger away from the stove. All in less than a twinkling.

The entire process of back pain works in the same way, with one exception. First you have a cause, except instead of it being a hot stove, it's a torn muscle, a stretched ligament, a squeezed disc, or any innumerable other possible imbalances of this nature. The cause instantaneously alerts the sensory nerve fibers attached to the particular part of your back that is affected by the disorder. These sensory nerves, which are tied into your main nerve cables, flash the message to your brain. The brain pulls the alarm, so to speak, and lights start blinking, bells start clanging, sirens start screaming—Pain! Now your effector nerves mobilize as the brain shoots messages back to the source.

Except that in this case you can not lift the affected part off the stove. If you were to willfully leave your finger on the stove, your pain would increase and you would likely suffer burn damage, with all its separate and even more painful consequences. With your back, however, there is no removing it from the cause. The cause of your pain is imprisoned within your back. So the reflex to withdraw from the source of the pain, as in the finger-on-the-stove example, is compromised. What happens, then, is that the effector nerves, trying to help the afflicted part of your back recoil from the source of its pain, are stymied. This produces spasm and further pain.

Although I have oversimplified it, this is the basic process that occurs with back pain. There are hundreds of variations on this theme, but they all add up to the same thing—anything from mild discomfort to exquisite agony, depending on the nature, site and cause of the disorder, and also on dozens of other factors, including time, severity and the general condition of your back.

So much, then, for our general study of the back—its general anatomy and the general anatomy of back pain. I am sure you are anxious to press on so as to gain a better understanding of the specific causes of back pain.

In the next part of the book I'll discuss what causes back pain and take you on a trip through the thick forest of disorders, symptoms and treatments. I am certain that at some point along the way we'll come upon your particular problem. It's my hope that once you recognize it and gain a better understanding of it, you'll then be ready to put your back, if you'll excuse the pun, behind you.

Part II

The Causes and Treatment of Back Pain

5.

An Outline
of the Causes
of Back Pain

I said at the end of the last chapter that at some point along the way on our trip through the causes of back pain we would come upon your particular problem. In a way that's inaccurate because it implies that your problem is limited to a single disorder.

That's the trouble with backs. Your problem might have started with a single disorder, even something as innocuous as a slight muscle strain. But if you're reading this book because you've been experiencing pain—recurrent, chronic and sometimes downright torturous pain—ever since your first episode, then chances are that the problem in your back is no longer limited to a single disorder.

Does that sound alarmist and unnecessarily gloomy? Perhaps. But because I promised at the beginning to pull no punches, and since that is the way the back operates, I would be remiss if I tried to obscure or gloss over that fact.

This does not mean that your back *is* necessarily a bee's nest of disorders. But when it comes to the back, one thing usually leads to another, and if you've allowed your particular weakness to progress unchecked, the likelihood is that your present instability involves more than one thing.

Therefore, as we proceed through the thick and tangled forest of disorders that cause back pain, don't be surprised if you encounter more than one tree bearing your name. Re-

member that in any closely planted forest, the roots of the
various trees tend to intertwine beneath the ground.

What causes back pain? What sets off those nerve endings
that clang like Chinese cymbals in the pain receptors of our
brains?

Next to the question of how to get rid of back pain, which
we'll be dealing with in Part III of this book, the question
"What causes back pain?" is the one I am most frequently
asked in my practice. It's a question that all patients with
back pain ask me. Curiously enough, in the course of my
teaching duties, it's a question I often put to my medical students.

That situation often goes like this: I stand before a group
of third-year students in the medical school at which I teach
—about ten or twelve of them. We are having an informal
seminar in orthopaedic surgery and the topic for the next
two hours is (what else but) *Back Pain.*

The first question I ask, naturally, is: "What causes back
pain, gentlemen?"

As each student volunteers a cause of back pain, I write it
on the blackboard. After about ten or fifteen minutes the
blackboard is completely covered with my chicken scratches,
and if I had more room I could squeeze in a few more
possible causes. Usually the students are astonished by the
long list of possible causes of back pain. They have had no
idea of the innumerable and different things, some localized,
some from other areas of the body, that can cause problems
with the back. The causes run into the hundreds. The list is
almost endless!

Anyone who treats patients with back pain must know all
the potential sources of back trouble and know how to ar-
rive at the right diagnosis. But when all is said and done, you,
the patient, are the ultimate diagnostician—that is to say,
your aching back is what makes the diagnosis.

This chapter shall be a brief representation of that blackboard I have my students fill up. Only now, instead of listing
all the possible causes of back pain separately, I shall organize
them into eleven general groups of causes and try to give you
a broad overview of each group. In the following chapters in
this part of the book I shall go into each of the groups in
greater depth and detail, explaining for each cause the signs
and symptoms, the diagnosis, and the various medical treatments.

1. Trauma

Trauma in all its forms probably causes more loss of workdays and man-hours than all other ailments combined. Trauma is injury. This can be a sudden twisting injury to the lower back, a blow to the area, a fall from a height in which you have sudden compression of the bones and discs in your spine, a sudden strain when lifting a heavy object, or a number of other dramatic events.

All these events constitute *sudden* trauma. In other words, the injury results in an immediate painful effect. When I was blocked during that spring football practice many years ago, that was a sudden trauma.

On the other hand there are injuries and strains to the spine that are more subtle. Their effects take longer to develop and often are so gradual that the victim may well not even be aware that the trauma took or is taking place.

This is *chronic* trauma, a mild persistent injury that has a cumulative effect. This is probably what my father suffered from. And provided that you are not a victim of one of the specific diseases or defects enumerated further on, chronic trauma is probably what started your back problem.

What sudden trauma is, is obvious. But what, exactly, is chronic trauma? Chronic trauma is sleeping on a poor mattress for many years. Chronic trauma is sitting slumped in a chair in a position which produces continual strain on your lower back. Chronic trauma is continually bending and lifting with your knees straight, even if the object you're lifting is only a feather. Chronic trauma is driving a car long distances with your back in a poor position.

Chronic trauma is any recurring strain put on your back, however mild the strain may be. Chronic trauma occurs in most of your daily lives—many times during each day, day after day. The cumulative effects of chronic trauma eventually reach a point at which your back is no longer capable of withstanding them. That is the point when pain occurs, and the more severe the pain is, the more likely is the severity of the trauma-induced disorder.

2. Posture and Curvature

Many chronic trauma conditions derive from faulty posture—in fact this is the most common underlying cause of back pain. It is true that our backs have not kept up with the rest of us with respect to adapting to our upright position. The back is still the weakest link in the chain of body parts that runs from our head to our toes. Yet our spines and associated back structures *have* made progress over the last few hundred thousand years. Our spines have adapted, and are probably still going through a long, continuing period of adjustment, to our erect posture.

In our section on the anatomy of the spinal column you learned that the spine is a long, slightly S-shaped affair. There are, in all, four curves in the spine between the base of the skull and the coccyx. Of these natural curves, two bend toward the front of the body, and two bend toward the back.

The two natural rearward-bending curves of the spine are due to the shape of the spinal bones. The other two—the forward-bending curves—are brought about by the wedge-shape configuration of the intervertebral discs.

The curves that are due to the shaping of the bones, the rearward-bending curves, are also found in the spines of four-legged animals, so it would seem that these two curves derive from the time when we were quadrupeds. The two curves that are due to the shape of the discs, on the other hand, are of later origin, having been developed in the process of man's assuming his erect posture.

The bony structure of our spines has remained virtually unchanged since before we descended from four-legged animals. However, the changes which were necessary when man assumed the erect posture took place in the more adaptable intervertebral discs.

The rearward-bending curves of the spine, produced by the wedging of the vertebrae, are called the *primary* spinal curves. The forward-bending curves, produced by the wedging of the intervertebral discs, are called the *secondary* spinal curves.

The primary curves were brought about in the process of strengthening the spine of quadrupeds against the stresses and strains of life with a horizontal spine. When the vertical position was assumed it was necessary for nature to counteract these earlier curves with curves in the opposite direction, while at the same time ensuring strength for the spine in its new position. It has been calculated that the spine is sixteen times stronger, owing to the presence of its natural curvature, than it would be if it were perfectly straight.

The secondary curves, the ones that only man has in his

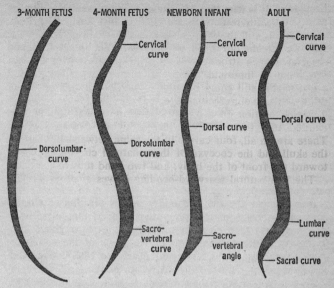

FIG. 8 Spinal curvature at four stages of life.

spine, are in the cervical region (at the top of the spine) and in the lumbar region (the lower portion of the spine above the sacrum). The cervical curve makes its appearance before birth, but apart from this a newly born baby's spine is similar to that of a quadruped. In fact, a young baby's thighs are, for a short while, flexed in the position in which a four-legged animal holds its hind legs, and it is difficult to straighten them out.

The lumbar secondary curve first makes its appearance when the baby begins to straighten out its legs. It becomes more marked when the baby sits up, and even more pronounced when the standing position is finally assumed and the baby begins to toddle. The effect of the efforts of a small child to balance itself when walking causes the curve to bow even more, but as the child becomes more sure-footed the curve becomes less acute. This is shown by the fact that a child's back becomes straighter and his bottom less prominent as he or she gets older.

The variation in the secondary spinal curves continues

throughout life. In early adulthood and in the prime of life
the secondary curvature of a normal spine is not very pronounced. In old age the tendency is for the lumbar (lower)
curve to become reversed, and the bend to the rear slowly
becomes a bend to the front. In other words, the back becomes bent with age.

In women the bow of the lumbar secondary curve is more
pronounced than it is in men. It is natural for a woman's
lower back to be more hollowed than a man's and for her
rear to be more prominent. This becomes even more marked
during pregnancy, when the lumbar curve increases to balance
the protruding abdomen. This increase in the lumbar curve also occurs in people of either sex whose abdomen is excessively prominent due to obesity, which in itself is a frequent
cause of back pain.

It is because the two secondary curves are due to altera-
tions in the shape of the intervertebral discs that these normal variations take place at different times throughout life.
If they were due to variations in the shape of the vertebrae
themselves, this would not occur nearly so easily, since the
vertebrae do not change their shapes normally.

Thus it is, then, that the spine, during the normal course of
its growth and development through the span of a single
human life, goes through normal changes in length and shape.

Unfortunately, it also goes through *abnormal* changes, especially in shape. These abnormal changes, most of which
are brought about by the effects of poor posture, change the
natural curvature of the spine, place abnormal stresses and
strains on its supporting structures—ligaments, tendons and
muscles—and result in back pain. Depending on the nature of
the abnormality the pain can be mild or severe. Usually it is
chronic, and each time it recurs it is likely to be a little
worse than previously.

Some curvature abnormalities are also produced by defective spine development. The contour of vertebrae may be irregular. Segments, or even entire vertebrae, may be missing.
Occasionally an individual might be born with an extra vertebra, which upsets the entire arrangement and balance of the
spine.

The consequence and significance of all these spinal abnormalities, whether brought about posturally or through
spinal defects, means that the spine is no longer able to properly do the job it was designed for.

3. The Slipped Disc

The "slipped disc" provides probably the greatest fascination, as well as the severest agony and most frequent debility, for victims of intense low back pain. Although it is true that many back pain victims have or have had disc problems, this still is not the most common cause of back pain. The disc *is* the source of most of the myth and ignorance that is bandied around about back pain, however.

A "slipped disc" neither slips, nor is it a disc. But because we are all used to the term "slipped disc" by now, we'll continue to use it in its generic sense. The condition popularly known as "slipped disc" is in reality a complete breakdown of an intervertebral joint in the spine, for that's what a disc is.

As with the other general causes of back pain I am listing in this chapter, I'll get into disc problems in more detail further on. Let me say for now that of all the backaches you can get from what we call an instability of the spine, the one you get from a damaged disc can be among the most agonizing. Conversely, just because you have a serious case of low back pain, don't automatically jump to the conclusion that you've got a "slipped disc."

Although not the most common cause of severe back pain, faulty discs are by far the biggest source of *serious* back trouble from a percentage standpoint. Along with those cases definitely identifiable during diagnosis as disc problems, there are innumerable problems that are traceable to the disc but are not yet far enough developed to show up as such. This is why it is so important that you start looking after your back once you've had your first episode with pain. Most severe disc problems, the ones that end up on the operating table, got that way because they were neglected in their early stages.

As often as not you can get along fairly well for a time with a slight disc disorder, provided it's slight enough. But only an early diagnosis can prevent it from progressing into a surgical condition—so long as the diagnosis is accompanied by a proper therapy regimen and so long as you follow that regimen.

Disc trouble can be found in patients of practically any age up to seventy or more, but most often it turns up in men in their thirties and forties. I know of no case of a child under ten ever having had a slipped disc; there have been relatively few teenagers so afflicted.

Nevertheless, although disc problems often are the result of acute traumatic injuries, they often also evolve from the chronic trauma that poor posture and sloppy habits, learned in childhood, inflict on the back.

4. Congenital and Developmental Defects

Although the entire process of conception and birth is amazing for its complexity and frequent perfection, errors do sometimes occur which leave newborn babies with anatomical defects. Quite often these defects are related to the spine and are a direct cause of back pain, disability, even deformity. Other pain-producing abnormalities may develop after birth during the early years of childhood and, if unattended, will eventually plague an individual after he has grown. Although a few are not, most of these spinal defects are treatable and manageable, and the pain they produce can be controlled.

5. Infections and Tumors

Since the back is alive with cells and blood vessels, it is susceptible to infections—that is, localized infections of the bones and spine. I am not talking about the old-wives' tale of the "cold in my back." I am talking about a serious infection of the vertebral bodies. These infections are relatively rare, but can occur as a result of direct implantation of bacteria into the bones. Or, the bones may become secondarily infected due to the infection of a neighboring kidney, uterus or prostate gland.

Any infection of bone is called *osteomyelitis*. When the infection involves the spine it is called *spondylitis*. Different types of bacteria can be the causative agent for such an infection, but *staphylococcus* is the most prevalent germ.

Not too many years ago *tuberculosis* of the spine was very common—in fact, the spine was the most frequently victimized of all the bone structures in the body by tuberculosis. Today, although rare, tuberculosis still does occur.

Another dreaded infection that can cause back pain is *meningitis*, an infection of the spinal cord itself. Naturally, when the spinal cord and its nerves are inflamed by infection, all the muscles supplied by these nerves will be in spasm and considerable pain will result.

The one cause of pain—any pain—a patient fears most is tumor. Our entire population has been alerted to the seriousness of cancer and of the relationship of this dread disease to pain. Subsequently, when an individual experiences recurringly severe back pain and seeks medical attention, one of the reasons many do so is to find out whether she or he might have cancer of the spine.

Fortunately, primary cancers, or cancers arising in bone, are relatively rare. More fortunately yet, the spine is an even less common site of primary bone cancer.

However, many other types of cancer which begin elsewhere in the body can either cause pain in the back through the phenomenon of what we call "referred" pain, or else can eventually spread to the back themselves, also causing severe and recurring pain there.

Not all tumors are malignant. Some just grow locally, and although they will cause some pain they do not spread. These are benign tumors. Tumors, both malignant and benign, may occur in the spinal cord. These of course will produce quite intense pain as they enlarge and involve the nerves.

6. Arthritis

Arthritis, by definition, implies involvement of the joints. The "itis" on the end literally denotes infection, but in the common use of the word today infection is not implied unless preceded by the word "septic." In other words, *septic arthritis* means joint infection, but *arthritis* by itself means an inflammation in the joint.

There are three types of arthritis which may involve the back and cause severe and recurring pain. (These are not limited to the back; they can involve almost any joint in the body.) *Osteoarthritis* is the most common of these. This is the arthritis that comes about by virtue of good old wear-and-tear. Simply put, what happens is that the surfaces of the back joints slowly wear out and cause stiffness.

Rheumatoid arthritis and its variants are actually diseases which involve the *synovium* (the lining of the joint). The synovium proliferates and destroys the localized joint cartilage. This leads to the ultimate destruction of the joint and, in the case of the spine, a growing together or fusion of the vertebral bodies. If you can imagine the pistons in the engine of your car expanding in their cylinders and then binding, unable any longer to move, you'll have an idea of how spinal rheumatoid arthritis works.

The third type of arthritis is much rarer than the first two. It is *gouty arthritis*. Most of you are familiar with the classic picture of a stout old man, looking somewhat like Benjamin Franklin (who did have gout), with a swollen big toe and a painful grimace on his face. He had a bad case of gout. Gout is not solely a disease of the rich, as it's often claimed to be. It afflicts everyone. It is a metabolic disturbance in which small crystals of uric acid are deposited about the joints. This causes a great deal of pain when it involves the intervertebral joints of the spine—plain old excruciating back pain.

7. Systemic Diseases

A systemic disease is one which is not localized in any one particular area of the body. It involves the entire system— thus the word "systemic." Many of you have had the so-called "grippe" or flu and have suffered not only the ravages of having your gastro-intestinal system assaulted at both ends, but have also suffered fever, chills, raspy throat, headache, and back pain. This is the "ache-all-over" kind of feeling.

Other more serious systemic diseases can also produce back pain in the form of muscle cramps, inflammation of the joints, or involvement of the spine and its contents, such as in meningitis.

General *metabolic* diseases also lead to backache. Metabolic diseases are diseases that primarily have their source in our glands. Included in this group are *hyperthyroidism*, or hyperactivity of the thyroid gland; *hyperparathyroidism*, or hyperactivity of the parathyroid gland; *Cushing's syndrome*, which is an oversecretion of cortisone from our adrenal glands.

Certain vitamin deficiencies can produce systemic diseases and thereby pain in the back. A lack of Vitamin C produces scurvy and a lack of Vitamin D produces rickets. Either of these can cause back pain.

Even circulatory problems can be a cause of low back pain. Circulatory disorders have to do with a decrease in the amount of blood entering the lower extremities due to spasms in the arteries, *arteriosclerosis* (the narrowing of the arteries), or low heart efficiency. They also have to do with poor blood return from the lower extremities, as occurs in cases of severe varicose veins or in *thrombophlebitis*. Of course poor circulation is more likely to produce pain in the legs than in the back; but especially in arteriosclerosis and inefficient heart-pumping, pain often manifests itself in the back.

8. The Aging Process and Hormonal Changes

Growing old is the inevitable process of all living things. The spine, too, is affected. I have already mentioned that as we age changes in the disc structure of our backs begin to occur. Our discs gradually lose their fluid by a process of dehydration and desiccation, and begin to shrink and narrow. Although this is a natural process, and it happens to everyone, it does not mean that everyone will end up with a painful disc problem. Most frequently it is the person who ignores this process and goes on treating his back as though he were still a youthful Hercules who has problems.

Another aging problem is limited to women. Women who have passed through the menopause tend to lose the *collagen,* or protein matrix, of the bones in their spines. Thus the bone becomes thinner. This lessening of density shows up very clearly on X-ray. The condition is called *osteoporosis.* Medicine still does not understand the specific reason why this process takes place, but it is apparently related to the hormonal changes that occur as a result of the menopause.

Besides post-menopausal osteoporosis, elderly people, regardless of sex, develop *senile osteoporosis.* This condition develops slowly and is irreversible; however, it is mild in some, severe in others.

Although back problems caused by the aging process are often irreversible, they need not be a constant source of pain or disability. I have had many patients in their seventies and eighties who, although their spines showed the same deterioration as those of other older people, had very little in the way of back problems. These patients are invariably the ones who have, throughout their lives, taken care of the supporting structures of their backs, even strengthened them, so that their supporting structures, especially their muscles, were able to take up the work that their spines, because of geriatric deterioration, were no longer able to do.

9. Pregnancy

Although the back pain of pregnancy is really due to chronic trauma (chronic strain) resulting from poor posture, weak muscles and additional abdominal weight, I am listing it separately because so many women who first develop back pain during pregnancy continue to have it for the rest of their lives. There is no single group of people who cry, "Oh, my aching back!" with greater frequency than pregnant women. Fortunately I have a wife who listens to her doctor-husband, and she was able to go through two pregnancies without any back pain. Her success carries an easily learned lesson for any pregnant woman who wishes to avoid the back pain of pregnancy and the post-delivery complications.

10. Referred Pain

This cause of back pain is pain that originates in other regions of the body but manifests itself in, or refers itself to, the back. It often presents a diagnostic dilemma to the doctor.

In the early stages of pneumonia, for instance, before fever occurs, the patient's only complaint may be back pain. Men with prostate trouble often complain of low back pain. Women with tipped uteri often express their symptoms in back pain. Kidney diseases usually evince severe back pain. People with ulcers will frequently find their backs "acting up." These are only a few of the sources of referred pain.

The reason referred pain occurs is due to the interlocking network of nerves which I described in the chapter on the nervous system. If nerves from different areas use the same pathway to reach the brain, it is possible for the brain to become confused. Thus if the center of pain stimuli is in, say, a diseased prostate gland, because the prostate's sensory nerve pulses run along the same nerve root as some of the nerves which supply the lower back, the brain will often interpret the signal as emanating from the lower-back nerves. It will then send out effector nerve pulses to the muscles of that region for protection, and lower back pain will result. Because of the referred-pain syndrome, doctors treating back problems must be aware of all these outside causes of back pain and must be prepared to eliminate these causes through tests and other means when diagnosing back pain.

11. Stress, Tension and Fatigue

Last but certainly not least in our panoply of general back-pain causes we have the emotional stressful backache. This can be entirely psychological or, as doctors like to say, "psychosomatic." An individual develops pain in his back as a defense mechanism in a situation in which he finds he can no longer cope with emotional difficulties. In such a situation great tensions that develop within his mind translate themselves into fantasized bodily ills, and quite frequently these imaginary bodily ills manifest themselves in the form of severe backache. In some cases this becomes a useful device to the sufferer—he takes to his bed and thereby avoids or delays making a decision or dealing with his real problem. This, of course, is an exaggerated situation, but I have seen it occur with much more frequency than you might imagine. Actually, this type of back-pain sufferer has nothing wrong with his back. But the pain he feels is still real and must be treated. In such a case the treatment is directed not so much at his back as it is to the causes of his psychological stress.

There is another type of back pain that occurs with plain bodily fatigue, and this is also psychosomatic to a certain extent. When someone is under a great deal of stress, when he does not get enough rest and allows unalleviated tensions to build in his body, the result will often be back pain. You'll recall that I said before that the back is, for evolutionary reasons, the weak link in the chain of body parts between the head and the toes. Because of this, when tension and fatigue are allowed to build in the body the first place pain is likely to strike is in the back. The components of the back that are most affected are the back muscles. The muscles will themselves fatigue and will no longer be able to perform their supportive functions. Usually they will go into spasm, and these spasms will cause severe back pain—whether in the lower back, the upper back, or all through the back.

I'll have more to tell you about backache, stress and tension later on. Suffice it to say now that in the case of this cause of back pain, as well as for all the other general causes I have enumerated in this chapter, the degree of pain you experience as a result of your particular back disorder is almost directly relatable to the condition of your back and its associated supporting structures. With the exception of irreversible diseases of the back, which are relatively rare, and of permanent structural defects in the spine, which are also relatively rare, back pain should *not* be a problem for anyone who takes the time and trouble to understand his back. From such understanding will come the knowledge of how to control back pain, as well as the motivational reinforcement for controlling it.

I have given you eleven groups of etiologies (causes) of back pain. These groupings represent perhaps a hundred separate, but in many instances related, causes. It is a thick forest indeed. It is no wonder, then, that the diagnosis and treatment of back pain can be such a frustrating and complicated task.

Diagnosis and treatment starts with your first visit to a doctor—so, please, step into my office.

6.

The Doctor's
Examination

Many people are apprehensive about seeking medical attention. In some instances they feel their complaints are too minor. In other instances they are afraid to hear bad news. People will therefore generally not consult a doctor until they have a condition that causes them at least a fair amount of discomfort, and even then they'll do it grudgingly. Grudgingly because—well, in spite of the relief they expect to obtain, who likes to face the fact that they are destructible?

After a severe case of back pain strikes, you are likely to hobble into the doctor's office and wait your turn if you don't have an appointment, or get miffed about having to wait anyhow if you do have one. You will be in a foul mood from the pain, probably in a fouler mood from wondering about the time and money the visit is going to cost you, and in a fouler mood still from imagining all sorts of wild and depressing consequences of your visit.

All this amounts to what I can only characterize as fear. You fear the pain. You fear the probable financial consequences. Most of all you fear the possible medical consequences. This is strange territory for you—at least that first time you are forced into a doctor's office. You feel you are standing on the brink of some new, unknown but certainly unpleasant journey. You resist it with all your might. Yet by now the pain in your back is strong enough to overcome all resistance. You need relief, first and foremost.

Another fear you carry along with you is in the form of the question: "What is he going to do?" Well, there is no magic in what the doctor, in most instances an orthopaedic surgeon, does. In a logical and methodical manner—established by four years of medical-school training, a year of internship, four years of residency training, usually two years of military doctoring, and another few years of private practice—he will proceed to diagnose the problem, relieve the pain, and establish a program of treatment and therapy.

He does this first by obtaining a careful medical history and a history of the specific complaint that brings the patient into his office, then by performing a meticulous examination and by ordering, on the basis of the initial findings, the necessary X-ray and laboratory studies.

Every doctor has his own pattern and idiosyncracies in performing the above procedures. I will discuss my own pattern in general so as to give you an idea of what to expect when and if you are required to consult a doctor. I may vary my pattern slightly in order to determine unusual conditions; however, the general approach to the history, to the physical examination, and to the X-ray and lab studies in a patient with back pain is fairly consistent.

Your First Visit

Suppose you were to come into my office. You would lower your quivering frame gently and carefully into a chair opposite my desk, look over at me with a pained beseeching expression, and wonder why I'm not immediately injecting you with painkillers. The reason I'm not is because pain, as agonizing as it can be, is one of the best diagnostic aids a doctor has to isolate the source of your trouble. So when you go to a doctor begging for relief, don't think he's a bad doctor just because he doesn't alleviate your pain first thing. He's doing you both a favor by letting you squirm for a few more minutes while he takes your history.

The history is very important, and it's the first part of the treatment procedure. What I would attempt to do after you sat down would be to gather some general medical information about you, if it was your first visit, and obtain as much verbal information about your specific complaint as I could. I would want to know the exact location of your pain and whether it is localized in one area or whether it radiates to different places. I would want details as to how the pain first started, what might have caused it, the first time it occurred, and the frequency of your attacks since then. I would then ask you about whatever previous treatments you might have had, whether prescribed by a doctor, a chiropractor, or a next-door neighbor, and what the results of their suggestions were. What I would be learning in this history-taking part of our visit would enable me to get a line on the "exact" cause of your pain, what aggravates it and, especially important, what will relieve it.

After spending some time on the history of your pain, I would then inquire about the state of your general health and about any past illnesses or surgery. I would also ask about your family and try to find out if backaches were common in other members of your family and if there are any diseases in your family's history that might be inheritable. Finally, I would inquire into your occupation, your work habits, your social life, your psychological state of mind, and even into your sexual activities and habits. It might seem strange to you at the time, but all of these factors are important in the evaluation of a patient's back pain.

The Examination

Next would come the physical examination. I would ask you to step into one of my examination rooms, undress completely, and slip into an examining gown, which goes on backwards so that you are entirely covered in front but partially exposed in the rear.

The first thing I would do would be simply to take a look at your back while you're still in a standing position. I would try to determine whether your spine was straight or tilted to the side, and whether your overall posture was satisfactory. I would also note whether you were muscular or flabby, lean or excessively heavy. I would then ask you to walk around a bit —towards me, away from me, sideways to me—and note any abnormality that might appear in your walking pattern. All this time I would be watching for expressions of pain on your face so as to discover which walking or standing activities cause the pain. Such activities would naturally be related to the underlying cause of your pain.

I would then ask you to stand on your toes, then on your heels. This would help me to determine whether there is any weakness in the muscles associated with these activities. Next I would have you bend forward as far as you could, then backward and to the sides, noting any limitations you might have in these motions and determining whether any of these motions cause you pain. I would then approach you and palpate (feel) your back, searching for the presence of muscle spasm and also getting an idea of the tone and quality of your back muscles. I would also press down on your back gently to discover any local areas of tenderness.

I would next have you lie down on the examination table. First I would measure the length of your legs. It is not true that most people's legs are of different lengths. Quite the contrary—I rarely find any difference between the lengths of a patient's legs. However, if you were to have a discrepancy in the length of your legs of half an inch or more, this could certainly be the primary cause of your pain.

I would also measure the respective circumferences of your thighs and calves. Normally, the circumferences should be about equal. The dominant leg (that is, your right leg if you're right-handed, your left leg if you're left-handed), is usually slightly larger in circumference due to greater muscular development. If for some reason a nerve root is being compressed, however, the muscles on the affected side are likely to atrophy, or grow smaller.

Atrophy also occurs when muscles are not being used, or are not being used normally. For instance, someone with an arthritic hip who has no nerve or muscle abnormality in his leg may develop atrophy of the thigh muscles because he can not walk properly.

I would then evaluate the circulation to your legs by examining your veins and palpating the pulse in your legs. Good circulation to the lower extremities is always very important and the competent diagnostician will always test for it.

Neurological testing would come next. I would test your knee and ankle reflexes by tapping these joints with the percussion hammer, hoping to get normal involuntary reflex movements. These tests may not be taken too seriously by most back-pain sufferers, but I can assure you that they are very important in disclosing serious back problems. For instance, the reflexes are diminished (reflex movement is decreased) when the spinal nerve roots are compressed, such as by a herniated, or "slipped," disc. Similarly, the reflexes will show up as hyperactive or excessive when the upper end of the spinal cord is damaged, such as with certain infections or other diseases. So when you see a doctor come at you with a little hammer while you're already in a good deal of pain, don't think he's indulging sadistic tendencies. He's looking for very important signs, signs that will tell him a lot about your back.

I would next test your sensations for sharp as well as soft objects. Different nerve fibers respond to these two different kinds of stimuli, and what I would be doing here would be looking for some significant information about your nerve roots. Because each segment of your skin is supplied by different nerve roots of your spine, when sensation is diminished in a particular area that area will correspond to a specific nerve-root. By properly interpreting the signs, the site of your problem can be determined.

If you were an older patient, or if you suffered from arteriosclerosis, or if you were a diabetic, or if I knew you were a heavy drinker (these are all reasons a doctor goes to such an effort to elicit a complete medical history prior to examination), I would certainly test your vibratory sensations with a tuning fork. The tuning fork is struck sharply so that it hums, then is held against a prominent bone on the foot, ankle or knee. Normally a patient will feel the vibrations quite readily, but in patients with peripheral neuropathy or disease of the nerves themselves, this vibratory sensation is markedly reduced or absent entirely.

I might conduct other special neurological tests if I think such are indicated on the basis of what you have told me in the history-taking part of our visit, but the above procedures are the ones most usually performed.

The next steps in my examination would be done to look for and evaluate any signs of tension in the sciatic nerve and any muscle spasm in the lower back. While you're still on the table and lying on your back, I would ask you to stiffen each of your legs and raise them, one at a time, as high as you could. If you could lift each straightened leg 80 degrees or more off the table *without* any pain in your lower back, this would be a sign that your sciatic nerve—the nerve most often affected by lumbar disc troubles—is not involved in your problem. If, however, the sciatic nerve is under tension due to pressure or irritation, as the leg is lifted, the nerve is stretched and further irritated, and pain ensues. This is a clear sign of disc disorder. If I were to find that you had a limited leg-raising capability, able to raise one or both legs only a short distance off the table, I would immediately suspect a disc as the source of your pain. Patients with back pain associated with arthritis or simply with local strain and muscle spasms will have normal or near-normal straight-leg-raising capabilities. Certain other special conditions cause diminished straight-leg raising, and these I shall discuss in the appropriate chapters dealing with the causes and treatment of back pain.

Next I would test your hip motions to rule out any possible source of pain in that area. Then I would go to the "Double Thigh Flexion Test." In this test I would have you bend both your knees, press them together, and draw both your thighs simultaneously toward your chest. In patients with disc problems this position is comfortable. But in those patients who have pronounced low back strain and spasm, or have a specific derangement of the lower back, attempting to bring the thighs to the chest is this way would prove painful.

Before I asked you to turn onto your stomach I would palpate your abdomen in order to determine whether there was any tenderness or any swelling or distension in that area indicative of an organic disease. Once again, we must remember there are many different causes of back pain, and the only way we can make a proper diagnosis is to eliminate as many of the possibilities as we can.

Once you were on your stomach, I would again carefully look at and feel your back, noting any evidence of muscle spasm or asymmetry. I would probe the spine itself from the neck right down to the coccyx, feeling for any tenderness and noting its exact location. If this mild palpation produced no tenderness, I would repeat the procedure, this time pressing more firmly, adding some of my weight to my hands. If this were still not painful to you, I would then begin to percuss your spine, gently tapping the vertebrae. I would use my hand as a cushion, but would rap quite smartly, much like a dentist tapping your teeth with the handle of his instrument looking for an infected tooth. If there is any pathology or any other kind of problem in the spinal bones themselves, this percussion will produce pain in the affected areas. Percussion will not produce additional pain, however, if your problem were a routine muscle spasm or a herniated disc.

There are several other areas of the back where I might find local tenderness. These may be over the rear portion of the superior iliac spine and along the iliac crest. Both these areas are sites of attachments of muscles and ligaments and, because of that, often become sources of pain whenever these structures are strained or partially torn.

I would then palpate the greater sciatic notch in both of your buttocks. The greater sciatic notch is an anatomical area in the pelvis. It is through this notch that the sciatic nerve, plus other nerves and blood vessels, flow through the pelvis, pass into the buttocks and then descend to supply your lower extremities. When the sciatic nerve is irritated and I press on this area, it will produce pain. Obviously, the more irritated the nerve is, the greater will be the pain produced by my pressure. This test helps me to determine whether your pain is localized in the back itself or whether there is some component of nerve root compression or irritation behind your problem.

The buttocks themselves are quite important in any examination for back pain. Although we often tease about the buttocks being nothing but fat, they do contain, as you'll remember from your anatomy lesson, strong underlying muscles—especially the famous gluteus maximus. The tone of this muscle is important in telling me something about the condition of your back. I would have you contract your buttocks as hard as you can and hold the muscles tight while I palpated them. Normally, they should feel equally firm. But where there is sciatic nerve involvement, the nerves to this muscle can be compromised and the muscle loses some of its tone—that is, it becomes softer and more flabby. Again, this is one of the signs I would look for if I suspected a disc problem.

There is also a reflex test I would use on the muscles in your buttocks. This is executed by my placing one of my hands flat across the buttock and striking it sharply with my other hand. Were I to feel an involuntary reflex movement under my flat hand upon striking it, that would mean that the muscle is still in good shape and, even if there are other signs of a disc and nerve problem, that the problem is not too far advanced. This reflex is absent when the nerve to the muscle has become compromised.

With you still on your stomach, I would ask you to clasp your hands behind your back and then arch your back so that I could see the effect of extension on your lower spine. This is generally a pretty painful motion if you have a disc problem or if you are having severe lower back spasms, so I would caution you to carry out the movement very gradually.

Then I would lift each leg up individually, holding your buttocks down firmly with one hand and placing my other hand around your thigh as I raise it. This maneuver tests the lumbo-sacral joint area in your lower back and in addition places stress on the femoral nerve which goes down the front of your thigh. One of the purposes of my physical examination is to determine whether there is any involvement of this nerve in your condition.

I would also palpate the upper end of your thigh bone and around the hip joint to see if there are any localized areas of pain which can stimulate back pain but which might be the real source of your problem.

Once this routine outer examination is completed and I've begun to gain a closer acquaintance with your back, I would then proceed to give you a rectal examination. This is of singular importance in any general examination for back pain. If you were a man, I would be checking your prostate gland and lower bowel and rectal areas for any growths or swelling. If you were a woman I would be checking the position of your cervix, which can be palpated through the rectum, as well as for any growths or swellings. All of these, no matter which sex you may be, are often a cause of back pain. In addition, rectal examination is the only way to properly evaluate the condition of your coccyx.

X-Rays and Myelogram

Once the physical examination is concluded, I then have to determine what, if any, X-rays are needed. For most conditions, four X-ray pictures are usually sufficient, that is, four different views of the lower back. I'll want to have a front-back picture and a side picture of the overall area of your spine so as to get a good view of the positioning of its vertebrae and the alignment of the vertebral bodies, and also so that I can study each vertebra and intervertebral space and note any abnormality. In addition I would want two specialized closeup views of your lower two disc spaces. In these pictures I would again be looking for any abnormalities in the alignment or configuration of these lower vertebral bodies and would also be looking for any narrowing of the spaces between the bodies. When a disc has collapsed or has herniated, there will be some narrowing. This is not an entirely reliable sign of a collapsed or herniated disc, however. The fact that there is no narrowing or that there is very little narrowing does *not* mean that there is not a herniated disc present. Conversely, the fact that there *is* narrowing, which means a disc may be collapsed, does *not* necessarily mean that this is the cause of the pain.

If I were looking for a herniated or collapsed disc on an

X-ray picture I would not see it. The routine X-ray can not show this condition, it can only point to it or point away from it. The X-ray picture does give me a good idea of the condition of your spine, however, and helps me to rule out certain possible problems and consider others.

A disc problem can be seen on a *myelogram*, and if I were to suspect a disc in your case I might order one of these. A myelogram is a special study of the contents of the spinal canal. It's a procedure that's done in hospital. In the past the myelogram was considered to be a very serious procedure, productive of headaches and other complications. Today, however, the procedure has been so refined that it is routine, and most patients are surprised at the lack of discomfort and aftereffects associated with it.

A myelogram procedure goes, roughly, as follows: the patient is taken to the X-ray department of the hospital. Under local anaesthesia a hypodermic needle is inserted into the lower part of the spinal canal. Since the spinal cord ends at a higher level than the site of the injection, there is no danger of damaging the cord by inserting the needle. A small amount of the patient's spinal fluid is extracted for laboratory analysis. After the extraction of spinal fluid, a liquid dye material called "pantopaque" is inserted into the spinal canal. X-ray pictures are then taken. The pantopaque shows up on X-ray as having a different density than the other spinal materials seen by the X-ray camera's lens. The spinal canal, injected with nine cubic centimeters of pantopaque, appears in the picture as a dense, whitish column. When a disc is herniated, its bulge or protrusion makes an indentation into the column of dye in the canal and the indentation becomes visible. By looking at this indentation, and by moving the column of dye up and down and examining it at different angles, the radiologist, or whoever is performing the myelogram procedure, can determine whether or not there is a herniated disc and, if so, the exact spot at which it has occurred.

If the diagnostician happens to suspect the possibility of an abnormality in one of the vertebrae themselves, for instance a defect in their alignment or configuration, other views of the spinal bones will be taken. These usually are oblique views, that is, taken at angles, so that more of the vertebral bodies and their parts can be seen.

Now, I would not have you undergo a myelogram unless I was pretty certain that your back problem was traceable to disc involvement and wanted confirmation as to the specific site and degree of the involvement. And even if I required a myelogram in your case, this would not be done during your first visit to my office, although the initial routine X-ray studies would be done.

Laboratory Tests

While you were still in my office, however, I would want to initiate some blood tests to complete my evaluation of your back pain. Routine blood tests, such as *blood count* and *sedimentation rate,* would help to indicate the general status of your health and would point out whether or not there is an underlying infection possibly causing your pain.

Special blood tests, such as a *blood urea nitrogen* study, which provides information about your kidney function, and a *blood sugar* test, which indicates the presence of diabetes, would also be called for.

A *uric acid* study would help me determine whether a gout condition might be behind your miseries, and certain tests for arthritis would also be required. The routine blood count and sedimentation rate tests often help to determine the presence of arthritis, but there are other tests which are more specific for certain types of arthritis, such as the *latex fixation* test and the *C-reactive protein* test.

If I were to suspect the possibility of a metabolic disease, such as a thyroid condition or tumor, being at the source of your problem, I would order other types of blood tests to enable me to evaluate these possibilities.

The Results and Diagnosis

Once the results of all the tests are back in my hands, I am then ready to make a final diagnosis. Obviously, all during the course of my examination I would have been tentatively eliminating certain possibilities and admitting others, and I might even have told you that certain findings pretty obviously indicated a specific cause of your pain. But I would not want to make my complete and final diagnosis until all the results were in and I was sure in my own mind that no stone had been left unturned.

After reviewing all the pertinent points in your medical

history, your present symptoms, the positive findings of the physical examination and the results of the X-ray and laboratory studies, my task would then be to inform you of these findings and explain what they mean. At this time I would be ready to tell you rather definitely what you have and what you don't have, and advise you of the necessary program of treatment.

No one likes to go through surgery. Although surgery is often required for the correction of advanced disc disorders, most disc problems and the pain they cause can be kept under control purely through sensible therapy. Other structural causes of back pain, unless they involve structural defects, rarely require surgery in their treatment. However, the pain produced by these causes will not go away by itself, and if the causes are allowed to progress, they will usually result in advanced problems requiring surgery. And since we don't want to make narcotics addicts out of you by putting you on the endless treadmill of pain-killing drugs, the only other choice we have is self-administered physical therapy. In other words, instead of letting your back continue to tear down, we want to build it up. This is the surest way to conquer your back pain.

Try a Little Self-Diagnosis

When everything is said and done, it is your aching back itself that makes the diagnosis.

What you tell your doctor in answer to his questions, the results of his own examination and of the X-ray and laboratory studies he orders, and several other considerations all serve to establish a diagnosis. To a considerable degree, the more accurately and succinctly you can describe your symptoms to him, the more quickly will he be able to get at the root of your problem and begin treating it. The inability of most patients to explain clearly what bothers them is a long-standing source of grief to modern doctors. Part of that inability comes from reticence on the part of the patient—reticence that derives, more than anything else, from fear.

Most patients are afraid to talk about their symptoms. This is the "bad-news" syndrome at work again. They figure if they simply keep their own counsel and say no more than that "It hurts!" somehow nothing bad will happen, or at least the bad news will be delayed.

Nothing, of course, could be sillier or more self-defeating. Doctors are not miracle workers. Surely, sooner or later, they'll get at the problem. But the longer it takes, the longer it will take the patient to get well.

Let's talk about your symptoms for a moment and see if we can't get you to be a little more helpful to your doctor if and when you are required to consult him. If he's the kind of doctor you should have, he'll bless you if you've been able to think out the answers to some things he'll want to know beforehand.

Consideration of your case begins with the aforementioned history, which means anything and everything you can tell him about your situation from the very beginning of your time on earth. Don't hold back anything, because with every fact you give him your true diagnosis becomes more evident. Indeed, with enough facts, your diagnosis becomes unmistakable. Accurate diagnosis is as much, if not more, a matter of determining what you haven't got as what you have. It is, simply put, a process of elimination.

The most likely causes of your back disorder are back strain (trauma), a compromised disc, or arthritis, in that order. To some extent each of these conditions displays one or more characteristics easily identified by you before you ever see the inside of a doctor's office. You can check these out yourself before you talk to your doctor.

For instance, if your pain is usually one that throbs away at a fairly constant nuisance level until a motion of some sort really gives you a wallop, you've more than likely got a case of severe low back strain. A symptom of this sort likewise pretty well rules out a disc.

Or, your pain may shoot down one leg or the other, or both. If it does, you can be fairly certain you've got disc trouble.

With regard to arthritis, the indications are also clear. If that's your trouble, you can't help noticing that it's worse in the morning. You wake up with your backache. It's not what you'd call an excruciating pain, but nevertheless it hurts, and bending over to tie your shoelaces is a tough proposition. Straightening up again is even tougher. The only pleasant thing about it is that in an hour or two you'll limber up somewhat, provided you keep on the move, and the pain will diminish or vanish altogether until fatigue sets in. But sitting still for long periods of time will kick up the fuss in your back again. That's arthritic pain.

I'm not giving you this little exercise in self-diagnosis in order to make you an expert on your back pain or to do away with the need of a visit to your doctor. I simply want to emphasize some of the things a doctor looks for when he asks you about the history of your back pain and how important it is for you to be able and willing to describe your symptoms accurately. Although a competent doctor will insist on using all the diagnostic aids at his command and will certainly not jump to conclusions about your condition until all the facts are gathered, it is enormously helpful to him if he can get a good history from you. He doesn't want to wait until the results of the lab tests or possible myelogram studies are ready before he begins to treat your pain, so he'll make a pre-diagnosis in order to get pain-relief treatment going right away, pending final diagnosis. With a good history and a careful physical examination, as outlined earlier in this chapter, ninety-nine times out of a hundred the doctor will have nailed down your condition before you've left his office. But remember, for him to do that, he needs your help.

7.

Trauma

The words "He broke his back" fill people with dread and arouse images of someone paralyzed and confined to a wheelchair. Severe injuries to the spine certainly can cause paralysis of the lower half of the body if the injury involves the spinal cord at the upper lumbar or at the dorsal (mid-back) levels. And if the cervical or upper section of the spinal cord is involved, paralysis of the arms can occur as well.

You might recall that Roy Campanella, the famous catcher for the old Brooklyn Dodgers, had his career cut short when he sustained a fracture of his cervical spine in an auto accident. This resulted in paralysis not only of his lower extremities but also of a good part of his upper extremities as well, and he has been confined to a wheelchair ever since.

A spinal fracture of this intensity can indeed be frightening —life-threatening as well. It is the most serious form of acute trauma and calls for immediate medical attention. Fortunately, in contrast with milder and more chronic instances of trauma, this sort of injury almost exclusively occurs in the context of a violent accident. It is not likely to be self-inflicted, unless, of course, someone is trying to commit suicide.

A less life-threatening, but still severe form of acute trauma is the fracture of a vertebral body or its segments. The term "broken back" is sometimes used to describe this type of injury, but what the term really refers to is a fractured vertebra. Such fractures most frequently occur as a result of falls from heights and automobile accidents, but even slipping on a banana peel or an icy sidewalk can produce them.

No matter the cause, the victim has immediate pain at the point of the fracture and, depending on the severity of the break, is unable to move or stand. When the fracture is slight or incomplete, the victim may be able to get about, although with considerable pain and difficulty.

Obviously the production of such acute pain after such a sudden injury will provoke a call for a doctor. Any doctor who sees a patient after such an injurious episode, with its attendant pain symptoms, will immediately suspect a fracture and take the necessary measures to confirm it. The patient must be handled with extreme care to avoid further injury and possible damage to the spinal cord and nerves before other examinations and X-rays are performed.

A problem in the diagnosis of spinal injuries may occur in the case of the patient who has sustained multiple injuries. In the evaluation and treatment of other injuries, the injury of the spine may be entirely missed, and this does not bode well for the normal recovery of the patient.

I recall an incident when I was a young resident in orthopaedic surgery which embarrassed me mightily but taught me a lesson I would never forget about covering all the bases in an examination. A middle-aged housewife, taking some curtains down from a window in her living room, slipped off her step-ladder and fell. Like the proverbial cat she managed to regain her equilibrium in mid-air and landed on her feet. Not her feet, really, her heels. After her heels hit the floor she crumpled onto her side, and her back appeared to have avoided the usual consequences of such a fall. Her first sensation was that of severe pain in her heels and then of some mild pain in her lower back.

She lay on the floor, unable to get up, and soon crawled to her phone and called her physician. She was eventually taken to my hospital's emergency room where I was called to examine her. She complained bitterly about her heels and when I examined them it was obvious that she had fractured both of them—there was already swelling and tenderness, and when I palpated the heels I could feel the crackling of the broken bones as they moved.

She also complained about her back and when I examined it the pain and tenderness seemed to be localized in the lower lumbo-sacral region. Her neurological examination was normal, so I ordered X-rays—of her heels and feet and also of her lower back. The X-rays of her heels revealed severe fractures of both *calcinei* (heel bones), whereas the pictures of her lower back showed no evidence of fracture or any other serious condition. So I ordered the appropriate treatment for her heel fractures and calmly dismissed her back pain as nothing more than a mild strain, certainly to be expected from the nature of her fall.

Later that day the attending orthopaedic surgeon examined the patient. We discussed the case and the type of heel fractures the woman had sustained, and then he said, "Do you have an X-ray of her lumbo-dorsal spine?" I looked at him and said, "No, she didn't seem to have any pain there."

He very carefully turned the patient onto her side and pressed gently on the area of the 12th dorsal and 1st lumbar vertebrae. The woman immediately winced with pain. I looked at the surgeon in surprise. Thereafter, when we had obtained the necessary X-rays of the region, we saw that there was indeed a compression fracture of the 12th dorsal vertebra.

The surgeon had a smile on his face when he turned and told me that such a fracture was very common in such falls as the housewife had taken. When people land with a heavy force flat on their heels, aside from the expected heel damage, the force is transmitted up along their legs and through their lower pelvis and lower spine to that part of the spine that is immobile—the part that is connected to the rib cage. The force puts a severe flexion pressure on the lumbar spine—the movable part of the spinal column. This sudden force is resisted by the immobile part of the spine directly above the lumbar spine and the result is often a compression fracture of one of the vertebrae at the junction of the two spinal sections.

Fortunately my ignorance and false assurance did no harm to the patient, but it was a lesson I never forgot and is something I always teach my students very early in their training—never fail to touch all the bases, whether you're doing an emergency examination or a leisurely one.

Whenever a fracture of one or more of the spinal bodies does occur, regardless of the severity, the patient should be admitted to the hospital where, after examination and X-rays determine the type and severity of the fracture, a program of treatment and therapy can be immediately started. (The one exception to this concerns a fracture of the coccyx, a painful condition but one which can be treated at home.)

Simple compression fractures of vertebrae—that is, the compression of the bone until it is crushed together—can be treated with bed rest alone for about ten days to two weeks or until the pain and spasms have subsided. A spinal support brace or neck brace should then be used for three or four months until healing is well advanced. Exercises to strengthen the abdominal and spinal muscles are then instituted.

In younger individuals who have considerable bone compression, a Plaster of Paris body jacket may be required. This is usually applied after the acute phase or when the pain and spasms have subsided. The body jacket is not, like a support brace, removable, but it gives better support and stability to the spine. It generally allows a younger person to be more active, yet prevents him from further injuring the damaged area.

Fractures of the transverse processes or of the spinous process of a vertebra (you remember these) are also very painful, but their treatment is a little less constricting. Simple bed rest and medication until the pain subsides is all that's usually called for, then gradual strengthening of the back muscles through exercise.

Sudden Trauma and Muscle Spasm

You'll recall that in Chapter 5 I divided trauma into two categories, *sudden* and *chronic*. The kind of trauma I've described so far might be characterized as *sudden acute* trauma, but since it's the kind that will usually get a doctor onto the scene immediately and will require a long and arduous recuperative period with some hospitalization involved, a detailed discussion of these injuries is really beyond the purpose of this book.

What is central to the book's purpose is the kind of sudden trauma that will not necessarily get you into a doctor's office, at least not immediately, and that you will tend to try at first to overcome yourself.

These are the sudden injuries to the back which do not result in fracture but do result in the tearing of muscles or ligaments or the partial or total rupture of an intervertebral disc. I shall devote an entire chapter to the problem of discs a few pages on, so let me for the moment talk about sudden trauma to muscles and ligaments, which is the source of back pain for so many of you.

All structures have a breaking or tearing point, and this holds true of muscles and ligaments. Lifting too heavy an object or load can cause tears in the muscles. Sudden and forceful twisting or bending motions can tear muscles and ligaments alike. Sometimes just bending the wrong way to pick up a dropped coin can exert an overstressful force on a fatigued or flabby muscle resulting in acute strain.

The hallmarks of these sudden traumas are immediate pain and spasm, both of which can be quite severe and disabling.

Now, you've seen this word "spasm" scattered throughout the book and you're probably curious to know a little more about it. So far, you might easily suppose that backaches are largely caused by defects of one kind or another in the spine or pelvis. This is not necessarily true. Anybody with an absolutely perfect spine from a structural standpoint shouldn't feel smug about it. Such a desirable state of affairs is no guarantee at all of immunity from back pain, because the general muscular setup of your back is also a leading performer when it comes to your aching back. And that brings us to spasm. Enough is known about spasm to fill a whole book, but for our purposes a few paragraphs will suffice.

Except as a word we use for a particular purpose, spasm doesn't mean much as such, and to say a person is suffering from muscle spasm is just about as informative as saying he is suffering from a cough. Strictly speaking, the word spasm, as applied to a muscle, merely describes a condition in which the muscle in question becomes acutely, convulsively and involuntarily rigid. Muscle spasm is a part of all injury—if you are hurt in any significant way, you'll experience spasm.

Such spasm is natural, and within limits it's a very valuable thing indeed. Before doctors came along, muscle spasm was just about the only protective measure available to nature in her effort to offer some aid to injury.

All muscles of your body, the big ones and small ones alike, voluntary or involuntary, have only one prime function—they contract. They contract for specific purposes and their contractions are governed by your brain through your nervous system. Brain-nerve-muscle—this process is indeed what enables us to exist.

The thing called spasm is nothing more than such ordinary brain-controlled contractions gone wild. If spasm strikes the muscles of the coronary artery—the one feeding the heart itself—we call it angina pectoris. If the involuntary muscles of the gastro-intestinal tract go into spasm, you've got colic, spastic colitis, enteritis, cholecystalgia, or any other fancy name you might hear your doctor use to describe a bellyache.

When enough irritation of any kind hits one of your voluntary muscles, the same spasmic contraction occurs. Such spasm in the muscles of the back, usually induced by sudden overloads or direct violent trauma, is a certain, if secondary, source of back pain.

In spasm, these muscles have taken matters into their own hands. Without specific orders consciously transmitted by your brain, they've decided to stiffen up in response to a demand made by nature. This spasmic, uncontrollable contraction process, undertaken in defiance of the supreme control of your brain, is fixed, set and rigid. No matter what orders your brain may send down to the muscles to relax or calm down, the renegade muscles, firmly locked in spasm, stay put. Knotted and strained, they soon begin to hurt.

A clumsy twist while balancing on a ladder, an awkward pirouette in a discotheque, or a pratfall on an icy sidewalk may wrench or suddenly stretch one of your back muscles beyond its normal limit. If the wrench is severe enough, the muscle will probably even tear. Or a ligament may rupture. Or a disc may even compress. This is sudden trauma.

Immediately all your surrounding and nearby muscles get themselves into a kind of physiological sympathy strike with the injured or traumatized tissue. They tighten up and begin to contract spasmically in an effort to protect the damaged part from further insult. This reaction is commonly designated as splinting. Sustained for too long a time, it produces more severe pain than the original injury.

It may or may not come as some relief to you to know that when you have spasmic back pain of this type it is only a symptom. But you'll be feeling much better much quicker if your doctor is able to spot the underlying cause of the spasm.

Spasm is not solely a symptom of sudden trauma. It operates with chronic trauma, spine-structure injuries or abnormalities, diseases of the spine and back, and referred pain. But since sudden trauma is such a frequent source of back pain I have included a description of it here because it's the single most significant and immediate symptom in this type of back-pain cause.

If you were ever the victim of a sudden wrenching strain or other traumatic injury to your back and failed immediately to consult a doctor you most probably found that lying on a hard floor, on your back, helped to ease the pain, but that any movement caused an intensification of the pain. In some instances in this kind of injury bed rest and a regular dosage of aspirin for a few days will clear up the major symptoms—that is, the injury will begin to heal by itself—and you'll be able to resume your normal activities. But be warned —your back will never be the same again unless you take measures to compensate for the weakness created by the original injury.

Generally, sufferers of sudden trauma are unable to rest very well on their own and the pain. sooner or later, drives them to the doctor for medical treatment. After the examination and X-rays reveal the problem to be in the musculature and/or ligamenture of the back, the patient is placed on complete bed rest. If the pain is extraordinarily excruciating, the first stages of the bed rest will be in the hospital. In most instances, however, the patient can treat himself at home, and once the injury has healed, should immediately start on a program of back exercises to strengthen the muscles in his back.

Disease of the spine causes only a small percentage of back pain. X-rays will sometimes reveal "osteoarthritic" changes in the vertebrae, but these do not often cause pain. Rheumatoid arthritis, a much more serious ailment, causes pain and stiffness, but it is relatively rare. Other pathologies, such as tumors and tuberculosis of the spine, are even more unusual. Even disc trouble is not as common as one might think. The same is true of the mechanically unstable spine caused by congenital malformation or developmental anomaly. In short, the likelihood is that if you suffer from back pain your condition is caused not by organic disease, but by muscles that are weak, tense, fatigued or all three.

It is weak, tensed or fatigued muscles that permit most sudden trauma to lay you low. A strong, resilient back is much more able to withstand the pressures of sudden stresses and awkward movements than a weak back. So then, I can't emphasize too strongly that once the basic healing process has been completed after a sudden traumatic injury, you should embark on a program to rebuild your back.

Another form of treatment which is often used in relieving the pain of sudden trauma are injections of local anaesthetics like Xylocaine or Novocaine, often mixed with Cortisone preparations. Generally these are injected directly into the tender area or into the muscle which is in spasm. The object of the injection is to anaesthetize the nerves that supply the muscle so as to relax the muscle, slow down or stop the spasm, and diminish the pain.

There is one particular physician in New York, a very

well-known doctor, who has an extensive practice in the treatment of patients recuperating from traumatic injuries. He particularly believes in the use of these injections. I have found, however, that they have a very limited and often mis-leading use. I think they are effective only in the treatment of ligament injuries, and where there is mild, localized spasm. I do not believe that you can inject enough Xylocaine or No-vocaine into muscle to obtain complete relaxation. There are just too many different nerve endings in a muscle and it is impossible to hit them all individually. However, as I mentioned, in certain instances these injections can be helpful in the relief of pain, especially if the pain is localized in one specific site.

The use of heat and cold in the treatment of back trauma is another area of controversy. A dictum in orthopaedic surgery is that in any acute injury—whether a sprain, frac-ture or bruise—for the first twenty-four hours ice should be applied to the affected area in order to reduce swelling. After that, heat should be applied for the purpose of increasing local blood supply so as to resorb whatever bleeding or swelling has occurred.

Now, in the treatment of traumatic injury there is usually a large area of the back involved and some of the swelling, which will usually include internal bleeding if there has been a tearing of tissue, is very deep. It is unlikely that either the heat or the cold involved in this sort of treatment will pene-trate to the very deep affected layers of the back, as it must to be effective. So I place very little faith in the use of either heat or cold in the treatment of deep back pain.

Both ice-bag and heat-pad treatments can lull you into thinking you're obtaining some kind of therapeutic relief be-cause they desensitize some of the nerves that are responsible for your pain, but once you've removed them the pain will come back.

If the pain is purely spasmic and is close to the skin, ice treatments may serve, for first-time sufferers of pain, to relax the muscles involved and break the cramp, but with chronic sufferers this procedure is usually without any merit and all you are likely to achieve is a large puddle of water in your bed.

Muscle relaxants are generally overrated in their effective-ness. They function mainly as mild tranquilizers and in those instances where the pain is not too severe, they may be of some aid. But it has been my experience that muscle relaxants do not in any way affect the time that it takes a patient's symptoms to disappear or his back to get well.

I am not hesitant to use pain relievers, however, in the acute stages of any severe back pain. As we know this pain can be not only profoundly excruciating, it can also be disabling. I have often seen people develop reflex paralysis of the bowels due to the severity of back pain. Therefore, in the first twenty-four to forty-eight hours following a sudden or acute traumatic injury or strain, I do believe that the patient should get as much in the way of analgesics or pain relievers as is necessary to keep him or her comfortable.

Chronic Trauma

We have seen in Chapter 5 how many factors can separately or together contribute to back pain. Whereas sudden severe trauma is often the underlying cause of your first episode of back pain, what happens after that is usually a case of chronic trauma. Chronic trauma is nothing more than the continuation of an underlying cause, whether that cause be sudden injury, poor posture, glandular imbalance, disease, a deteriorating disc, or whatever.

Chronic trauma is the recurrent injuring or damaging of the site of your original cause of pain, plus the injuring or damaging of adjacent and dependent sites in the back. This is where the domino theory really comes into play. Once you've sustained your original injury or other cause of pain your tendency, once the original symptoms are relieved, is to relax your guard and return your back to its normal schedule of activities. But although the original symptoms may have been relieved, the original cause has *not* been cured.

These factors create a situation which gradually leads to a return of backache, perhaps starting at night after a long, tension-filled day, perhaps starting in the morning after a long period of inactivity. Discomfort will gradually increase over a period of time and will eventually begin to spread through your entire back or to your thighs and arms. Finally you reach the point where you are never comfortable. You "hold" your back in certain pain-relieving positions only to find that soon new pain starts as a result of your awkward posture. The whole process of pain is like an out-of-control forest fire, and no matter how many "fire-breaks" you build to contain the flames, they invariably seem to leap across the breaks or fan out in other directions. Often a sudden minor blow, a sudden innocuous twisting motion, a sudden stooping or lifting may trigger an attack of acute spasmic pain that will force you to go to bed or even put you in the hospital.

This is a generalized picture of how chronic trauma works. Sound familiar?

In a healthy person whose back is protected by strong, resilient muscles it takes a much more serious trauma to produce an attack of back pain. But the difference between injury to a healthy back and to a poorly conditioned one goes further—the otherwise healthy back recovers much faster under sensible and adequate therapy.

In the end, if you don't take adequate measures to prevent it, the chronic-trauma process will leave you in worse condition than the consequences of sudden trauma. This is because you have not only re-abused your original back injury, you have now injured, or weakened, adjacent components—to the point that your entire back is in a state of protest. It is weak, it is deconditioned, it is painful, and it is frequently debilitating.

Treatment is usually similar to that for sudden trauma —with an emphasis on bed rest, pain killers, muscle relaxants and so on. These may relieve the pain, but they surely don't cure your back.

There is an additional form of treatment that in the long run, without proper therapy, can be harmful and lead to even more problems. This is the employment of back braces and such.

The use of braces and other back support devices is rather extensive. In the instances of certain back problems they are absolutely necessary for proper healing of an injury. But the prolonged use of braces in the treatment of chronic back pain is plain wrong. It is like walking around on crutches long after your broken leg has healed.

Back braces and other supportive devices tend to further weaken the muscles which support the spine. In the long run, if you ever hope to solve your back pain, it is imperative that you have strong muscles and not let them further atrophy as a result of the inactivity braces require. Too many people unnecessarily come to depend on braces and other supportive devices, and the longer they wear them the longer they will need them.

In the treatment of fractures and occasionally after surgery, braces are necessary for the purpose of immobilization and healing. But the extensive use of braces in ordinary back pain, however severe, is foolish, and anybody who relies on them is deluding himself.

The only cure for a conventional bad back, *once the original cause is diagnosed and corrected,* is physical reconditioning. Analgesic injections, hot-and-cold treatments, diathermy, manipulation, relaxants, braces and the like are merely tools to relieve the symptoms of a bad back. The *only* tool for cure is the rebuilding of the back structures through exercise.

8.

Posture and
Curvature Problems

This chapter is probably the most important one you'll have read up to now. Most conventional back problems arise out of faulty posture and spinal curvature. It is these two factors more than any others that decondition the back—weaken the spine, its muscles and other supports—over a long period of time and make it that much more likely that both sudden and chronic trauma will occur.

Posture

Let's consider posture first. Posture is the position in which all your bodily structures relate to one another, whether you are standing, sitting or lying down. At the center of the relationship is the spine and its supporting structures.

If we stand and sit straight, our spines must be straight. If we slouch when standing and sprawl out when sitting, our spines will be excessively curved. Therefore the spine and posture are intimately interrelated.

A straight spine insures good posture. Conversely, good posture insures a straight spine. By a straight spine I do not mean a rigid, vertical pole. I mean that the spine will be set in the alignment and configuration in which nature, or the good Lord—depending on your persuasion—designed it for optimum function.

But what is good posture? I'm sure you can all recall your parents saying to you when you were young, "Stand up straight, get your shoulders back!" Is that good posture?

Not necessarily, because forcing your shoulders back will usually thrust your stomach out, and that's not particularly desirable.

Perfect posture would be an erect position of the spine, with only a minimum of curvature due to the natural spinal curves. Keeping these curves at their minimum does insure good posture because the straighter the spine is, the more evenly are the weights, loads and stresses distributed along the surfaces of the vertebral bodies. The distribution of weight determines the forces exerted upon the intervertebral discs and upon the vertebral bodies themselves.

Thus, if a person with good posture were to bend to lift a heavy weight, he would be much less likely to suffer a

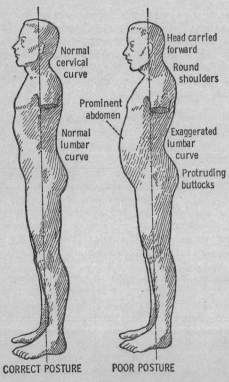

CORRECT POSTURE   POOR POSTURE

FIG. 9   Correct posture vs. poor posture.

traumatic injury to his back than the person with bad posture. This is simply because the person with good posture, in placing the unusual force on his back, distributes much more of the force throughout his entire spine, whereas the poor-postured person tends to localize the entire force in one area. Such is the fine line between injury and non-injury.

A simple law of physics states that when a force or weight is applied to a curved structure, the greatest stress is exerted on the concave or inner side of the curve. Therefore the more pronounced a curve in the spine is, the more uneven is the load of pressure over its surface, with the greatest loads concentrated at the apex of the curve. This in turn will cause excessive wear (a form of chronic trauma) on the intervertebral joints at the curve's apex, so that degenerative changes and the wear-and-tear factor will occur earlier than normal in the spine's life.

Compare the situation to an automobile's tires. When a tire's wheels are properly balanced and aligned, the tires will wear out evenly and will last for their natural wear span of 30,000 to 35,000 miles. However, if the wheels are not balanced, the tires' treads will wear unevenly and the tires will usually have to be replaced long before their maximum potential mileage is reached.

Unfortunately, we are unable to replace our spines, or portions thereof, when they begin to wear out prematurely. So it is imperative that we prevent premature wear by keeping all the parts balanced so that the weights and forces are distributed as evenly as possible. This is the only way we can keep the wearing-out process to a minimum and prevent premature spinal instability. Good posture achieves this goal.

People who are slouchy or round-shouldered will develop back pain sooner or later, more likely sooner, as well as osteoarthritis of the spine. People who stand with their shoulders back but have pronounced swayback, or increased lumbar lordosis, will develop low back pain and are very good candidates for further complications, such as disc disorders.

Posture is not only important when standing. Good posture embraces all positions of the body and is equally important when sitting, lying down, even when sleeping.

How do you establish and maintain good posture? Since you now have some understanding of the spine and how it works, all it takes is a bit of healthy motivation and self-discipline on your part. Good posture need not be a continually conscious concern, once you get it in your head that you are going to maintain good posture and avoid a host of potential back problems. It's mainly a matter of developing and maintaining the muscles which will hold you erect, until good posture becomes second nature.

First, good posture while standing consists of lifting your head as far away from the toes as possible, yet keeping your chin tucked in. This flattens the curve in your cervical spine. As you do this you should also make sure your pelvis is tilted forward by contracting the powerful muscles in your buttocks. This flattens the curve of your lumbar spine, and both simple maneuvers together place your spine in its most desirably erect position. By concentrating on these two simple things—head high with chin tucked in, pelvis forward— your spine automatically straightens and is prepared for the most even load distribution possible.

Naturally, when you first start to perform these maneuvers you will feel slightly uncomfortable and stiff, for your back is probably not used to good posture. But pretty soon you'll begin to notice a difference.

In fact, try it once—right now. Stand up, elevate your head with your chin in tight, then squeeze your buttocks and let your pelvis thrust forward. Hold it there for a minute— just freeze in that position. Feels different, doesn't it?

Continue to hold it and discover how you can almost actually feel your spine straightening out and the strange but not unpleasant sensations tingling up and down your back. Those sensations are, in effect, your spine coming awake. Now drop back into your regular posture and feel the difference. And you thought you had good posture?

Try it again. Hold it a little longer this time—head up, chin in, buttocks clinched, pelvis forward. Notice how your shoulders fall naturally back, instead of having to force them. Your parents had the right idea, but the wrong approach.

Still up there? Good. I'll bet if you had a bit of pain when you started reading this chapter you're finding that it diminishes while you're holding that good-posture position.

Hold it a little longer and enjoy the pleasant sensation as your back muscles relax and lessen the intensity of your ache.

All right, back to your normal posture again. There, you see? There *is* a difference, isn't there? After the effects of the good-posture position wear off you'll notice your ache return, along with all the other little signs of discomfort that come from your natural slouch. Do you see the point?

Good posture is not a difficult thing to achieve, even now. But the longer you wait to achieve it, the sooner you'll develop severe back problems. The little exercise I just gave you is something you should work on as many times as you can until the position begins to feel natural. I don't promise that by itself it will relieve pain, but it will surely make your back feel better and stronger, especially if you can eventually make the position your new, permanent standing posture. And it will go a long way toward preventing future pain.

In the life-long contest between you and your back, posture is practically the whole ball game. There is absolutely no substitute for good posture, and you can take it from an old sawbones who has suffered his own back pain—the achievement of good posture does more than anything else to prevent back pain.

Most trauma pain is caused by poor posture. Most, if not all, stress, tension and fatigue pain is caused by it. The same for disc pain, pregnancy pain and all other kinds of lower back pain. Upper back pain too—stiff necks, shooting pains across the shoulder blades, the whole bundle.

Test Your Posture

A good way to check your posture and also to learn how good posture feels is to test yourself against a wall. Start with your back leaning against the wall and your feet about twelve inches away from it. Bend your knees and lean your upper body forward so that your back is somewhat rounded and the only part of you that is touching the wall are your buttocks. Then begin, very slowly and gently, to raise yourself backwards against the wall so that you flatten each individual vertebra against it, starting at the lowest lumbar vertebra and gradually working up your back. As you start to press the mid-portion of your spine—the dorsal spine—against the wall you will notice that your lower or lumbar spine tends to pull away from it, so that you can actually slide your hand between your lower spine and the wall. Stop at this point and press your lower spine back against the wall. Concentrate on holding it there as you commence again to further straighten your upper back until your entire spine, from sacrum to neck, is firmly pressed against the wall. During this maneuver your knees have remained bent. Now gradually straighten your knees by pushing up from your lower legs and feet, but continue to keep your back against the wall. Once erect, push yourself away from the wall, maintaining a posture so that your whole body is in a straight line.

This may be a difficult test for you to do, but if you can master it you will get an excellent idea of what proper spinal alignment feels like. I'm not recommending a ramrod stiff back, the kind you only see, along with dueling scars, on Prussian officers. But good vertical alignment of your spine is an ideal to be sought with determination and self-discipline. It won't make a Prussian officer out of you, but it will give you all the benefits of good posture.

Good sitting posture consists of sitting on a firm chair with the small of your back snugly resting against the chair's backrest and your feet flat on the floor. Rather than leaning or settling backwards into the chair's cushion, it is better to lean slightly forward. This reduces the lumbar lordosis or so-called swayback tendency of your lower spine.

This same position is also desirable for driving a car. You should sit close to the steering wheel when driving so that it is not necessary to stretch your legs way out to reach the foot pedals, thus sagging your lower back.

Your sleeping posture is also of great importance with respect to the avoidance of back problems brought about by postural defects. A good firm mattress is a necessity, otherwise your body sags in bed and distorts the spine. Your spine will rest most profitably if you sleep on your side with your knees bent, or at least with one knee drawn up. Or else, sleep on your back.

Never sleep on your stomach if you can help it, because this causes a pronounced increase in the curvature of your lumbar spine and creates strains and tensions in your back muscles and ligaments.

For those of you who have a constant aching back a very comfortable sleeping position is with your head on a thin pillow and two or three pillows under your knees. The flexed elevation of your knees tends to flatten out your lumbar spine and reduce the strain on your back, thus relieving your pain.

Many of you have surely noticed that standing in one position for a long time produces lower and sometimes upper backache. The cause of this discomfort is due to the relaxing of the muscles of your abdomen and buttocks. This allows your frontal body features to sag forward, which increases the curvature of your lower spine and puts a strain on your back. If you have to stand in one place for a long time, a simple way to avoid this is to rest each foot alternately on a low stool. This tends to straighten your lower spine and relieves the stress. The footrest which is set into the bar at your favorite cocktail lounge is there specifically for that purpose. The longer a customer can stand comfortably, the more drinks he will purchase—and that's considered good business.

Whenever I perform surgery and the operation is lengthy, I always obtain a small stool on which to rest my feet, usually shifting from one foot to the other as necessary to relieve any stresses on my back. This little maneuver, carried out repeatedly and naturally during a three- or four-hour operation, has spared me many a sore and stiff back. I can actually operate more comfortably now than I could ten years ago—before I awoke to the cause of my "post-op aching back."

Posture during lifting maneuvers is often neglected. I am certain that no one has been taught to lift with their knees stiff, yet in a single day I see dozens of people lifting things in exactly that manner. The simple fact is that bending forward from the waist with the knees straight to lift anything causes stress at the lumbo-sacral region of your spine and can be very injurious. Naturally, the heavier the weight of the object being lifted, the more likelihood there is of something popping. One of the things I drill into all my back patients over and over again is that anytime they wish to get close to the floor, for whatever purpose, they must bend their knees. The feet should be separated and preferably one foot should be slightly ahead of the other. In lifting keep the object as close in to the body as possible in order to decrease the length of the leverage arm and thus further protect the back from strain. Never bend or lift from a rotated position. Always face the situation squarely.

These are just a few simple prescriptions on how to avoid the more obvious strains that careless posture or motions bring about, and on how to reduce the incidence of chronic trauma.

But my laying out these prescriptions is not enough. You've got to carry them through. In all my years of orthopaedic practice I have hardly ever had a back-pain patient who did *not* have bad posture. What's more, without exception every one of my patients who has experienced improvements in his condition has done it first through the self-disciplined pursuit of better posture, then through the building up of the back muscles through exercise regimens. The exercise therapy which I advocate to help you control and eliminate your back pain will not be half as effective if you do not at the same time retrain your posture. If you conducted the little back-straightening exercise I gave you earlier in this chapter you no doubt saw how proper posture changes the feelings you have in your back. This is an excellent exercise to do whenever you feel your back muscles begin to tire and your spine begin to sag, because it redistributes the forces and loads your spine has been bearing.

What you should now do is make that little exercise an increasingly frequent part of your daily routine. Head high, chin in, buttocks clenched, pelvis forward—the more often you do this, and the longer each time you hold it, the more time your spine and back muscles will be treated to proper alignment and load distribution. It should eventually become as second-nature to you as moving your bowels or brushing your teeth.

There are many reasons for poor posture, and most of them can be chalked up to pure and simple laziness. Certainly there can be congenital spinal defects or disease-induced causes, but these are rare in most cases of ordinary back pain. (I will cover these in succeeding chapters.) The vast majority of you have your back pain simply because of poor posture and the complications this condition eventually brings about.

Most poor posture habits develop and solidify in childhood. Perhaps the most significant reason for this is that parents constantly nag their children to "stand up straight" or "stop slouching" or "stand like a man." Such directives from parents to children are fraught with danger.

First, anyone who knows anything about the psychology of children knows that most youngsters tend to do the opposite to what they are told—especially when what they're told is delivered in the form of nagging complaints and the like. So children, or most of them, secretly rebel against such an approach.

Secondly, children are usually quicker to spot hypocrisy than anyone else, and when they're told to stand up straight by a slouching parent who himself is not standing up straight, they tend to become cynical about the propriety of such advice.

Third, youngsters gain many of their character traits and habits through imitation of their parents. So the parent with bad posture will most likely have children with bad posture, no matter how many times or with what intensity the parent keeps after them. Most people I know who have straight backs have children with straight backs. Unfortunately, they're astonishingly few.

Fourth, most parents who attempt to "teach" their children good posture, no matter how commendable their motives, usually haven't the slightest idea of how to go about it and often fill their kids with more misinformation than information. For instance, to order a child to throw his shoulders back and keep them there is not informed teaching. Every time I see a youngster react to such a command the shoulders are thrust back until the shoulder blades are practically touching, but the head continues to hang forward like that of a bird reaching for a worm. "Chest out-stomach in" is really not the right way of going about it either, for although it takes in two of the components of good posture, it ignores two others—the position of the lower back and pelvis, and the position of the neck and head.

Good posture does not begin with the shoulders, chest or belly. It begins with the head and the pelvis—once they are straight, everything else will fall into line.

Aside from their nautral rebelliousness, children also have other aspects of their own psychologies working against them. Some children, usually boys but sometimes girls too, grow very fast. They shoot up until they begin to tower over their contemporaries. This often induces self-consciousness, and a sort of permanent slouch results as they try to appear less conspicuous. Sadly, they usually don't get very much understanding from their parents on this score, especially because their parents are delighted to see them growing so tall and healthy. Thus, between the taunts of their shorter peers about being so gawky and the naggings of their parents to stand up straighter, psychological chaos results. Since this usually occurs at a time in a child's life when he is more concerned with peer-group approval than parental approval, and since it happens at a time when the child is at his or her most rebellious —the pre-teen and early teenage years—the slouch is favored over erectness, and soon becomes permanent.

A similar psychological phenomenon is common to young girls. I have often treated women with poor posture and severe back disorders stemming originally from poor posture.

Almost without exception I find, when taking their histories, that as young girls, during that period when their breasts were forming, their deep-seated embarrassment over these unaccustomed appendages caused them to hunch their shoulders and round their backs in an attempt to hide this development. Since the process of breast development takes a few years, they had plenty of time to develop poor posture and they tended to carry that posture with them into adulthood.

As a sidebar to the breast-development story, let me also say that the sagging-breast anxiety which so many women agonize about is partly due to their poor posture. Next time you go to a nudist camp compare the number of sagging bosoms to the number of slouched chests and rounded backs. Then compare the number of firm, upstanding bosoms to the number of straight, erect backs. I'll bet you the price of this book that you won't find one full, high bosom attached to a rounded and curved back.

In this connection, here's a story that might amuse you. Several years ago an attractive woman in her mid-thirties was referred to me because of prolonged, persistent pain throughout her upper back. The cause of her pain had thus far evaded diagnosis. She had already seen several doctors who had given her heat treatments, injections and various types of pills. But there had been no relief. Chiropractors had manipulated her neck, shoulders and back to no avail. She had no history of injury or illness that would appear to be productive of back pain. She was an active woman who played tennis and liked to swim, but now felt that she could no longer pursue these activities. Examination revealed that she was a very thin woman who appeared to be in good health, although she was obviously tense. During my examination, as I had her do some bending movements, she mentioned that it was her plastic surgeon who had referred her to me. I looked at her questioningly and asked why she had been to a plastic surgeon. She then told me that two years before she had undergone silicone injections in both her breasts in order to increase their size and improve their shape. At this point she pulled her gown away from her shoulders and exposed two very large breasts. Suddenly I realized why she was having such pain. This woman, who weighed ninety-eight pounds, had breasts big enough for a one-hundred-fifty-pound woman. She just did not have enough muscle strength in her shoulders and upper back to support them. Consequently her muscles would fatigue and she would constantly slouch into poor posture. The solution of her problem was easy. No, I did not suggest that she have the silicone removed. I started her on exercises designed to strengthen the muscles in her upper back and shoulders. It took her three months of diligent work to obtain the necessary muscle strength, but when she did her pain disappeared entirely. As far as I know, the pain has never returned.

Plastic surgeons specializing in silicone breast implantations to restore sagging bosoms would have a lot less business if more women, especially those who are worried about the esthetic configuration of their breasts, were to develop good postural habits in their early years. Orthopaedic surgeons would have less business too, and when it's a matter of back pain due to sloppy posture, I'm all for that.

Swayback

Perhaps the most frequent postural defect doctors encounter is *excessive lumbar lordosis,* or swayback, which is the most common cause of chronic back pain.

Simply stated, swayback is nothing more than the excessive curvature of the lumbar portion of the spine. The lumbar spinal curve, which I've already talked about, is without doubt the most critical of all the regions of the spine, for it is in this area that the great majority of back disorders occur. Lower back pain, as we've already seen, can be caused by many different factors, some separately, some operating in a kind of satanic unison. Not to be discounted in the symptoms of lower back pain is this peculiar, but not uncommon, problem.

It is usually shorter people who have the best posture. This is probably due to the fact that shorter people, just the opposite of prematurely tall folks, tend to stand up taller in order to psychologically compensate for their lesser physical stature. Thus, good postural habits are developed earlier in their lives. Additionally, shorter people have shorter backs and a lower center of gravity than taller people. They have smaller bones and generally have less weight, and therefore less back loads and stresses, to carry around.

Swayback is not a serious condition, and can easily be overcome with compensatory postural awareness. Yet if it's ignored it can produce various disorders, severe pain, or long-term discomfort. You'll recall that the spine is like a stack of blocks forming a column, with a cartilage cushion (disc) between each block. Coming out at the back side at each disc level are the nerves which supply the muscles and carry sensation. When this column of blocks bends forward, the back sides of each block are forced closer together. If the cartilage cushion holding each block apart gives way, it allows the back side of the blocks to come closer together, pressing on the nerves that come out between them. This pressure can cause pain and muscle spasm, and this is one of the results of pronounced swayback.

Remember also our guy-wire analogy of earlier. Guy wires in the form of muscles and ligaments attach to each vertebral block in the column of blocks that is our spine, holding the entire business in position. If the front guy wires (abdominal muscles) become lax, weak or flabby, they allow the lower back or lumbar curve to sag further forward, producing a swayback condition and the same strain problem described above.

If you have a swayback condition it means that you are unusually susceptible to lower back strain. If injury or repeated (chronic) stress to one or more lower back discs occurs, severe disability may result, with a painful spasmic "catch" in your lower back (lumbago) and intense pain shooting down one or both legs (sciatica). Between these attacks the back will probably be chronically sore, stiff and achy, with less severe attacks of "cricks" and catches (unstable lumbosacral joint).

Occasionally surgical procedures are required to correct backs of this nature, but more often conservative management can eliminate the pain. By "conservative management" I mean the institution of proper postural habits and exercises to strengthen the "guy wires". The foot-on-the-stool approach is also very helpful in swayback-pain management.

Dorsal Kyphosis and Scheuermann's Disease

Another postural problem comes from upper back stoop or slouch. When you grow up with that sort of habitual posture—shoulders well rounded (not the same as sloped prizefighter's shoulders), chest sunken, belly usually protruding—you set up a whole chain-reaction of possible disorders. You not only create an excessive bend in the dorsal curve of your spine (upper b⁻ck), you also increase your cervical (neck) and lumbar (lower back) curves.

When there is pain in the lower back there is likely, sooner or later, to be a similar strain in the neck. The cervical or neck curve is the matching component of the lumbar or lower back curve, and is subject to the same mechanical problems. The curve in between, the dorsal curve, which curves in the opposite direction, connects these two curves. If the dorsal curve becomes excessive, it accentuates the lumbar and cervical curves, and a whole new bucket of problems can occur, including neck "cricks," headaches, dizziness, shoulder-arm pain, and sometimes "crazy" feelings.

Pronounced round-shoulderedness not only produces or promotes swayback and ostrich neck, it can in itself produce pain and disorder in the mid and upper back similar to any of the other marked spinal-curve problems. These usually have to do with the vertebral bodies and the compression of nerves and discs. The condition is known as *excessive dorsal kyphosis* and its relief is best achieved through postural and exercise therapy.

Associated with excessive dorsal kyphosis is a thankfully rare condition known as *Scheuermann's Disease*. This is a rounded-back condition which is found almost exclusively in adolescent boys. But whether the disease is a result of poor posture, or poor posture is a result of the disease, we don't really know. It is painful and constricting, and can only rarely be relieved by surgery.

Scoliosis

Whereas all the conditions I've covered so far in this chapter relate to *posture,* which describes the anterior-posterior (front-back) configuration of the spine, there is one very significant and not uncommon condition that relates to *curvature,* which in medical parlance describes the spine's lateral (side-to-side) configuration.

Just as Scheuermann's Disease is found almost exclusively in young boys, this condition most frequently occurs in young girls. It is called *scoliosis,* and is a condition in which one or more regions of the spine assume a lateral bend or slightly S-shaped curve. Since the normal spine should be straight up and down when seen from the front or back, this is definitely an abnormality.

The cause of this deformity is still unknown, but if it is diagnosed early it may be corrected or prevented from progressing with the use of braces or body casts. If the curve progresses in spite of such treatment, however, or if the diagnosis is made too late for correction, surgical correction can be achieved.

Such surgery consists of straightening the spine as much as possible in the area of the abnormality, without damaging the spinal cord, and then securing the straightened-out part through fusion. (Fusion of the spine consists of connecting all the rear portions of the vertebrae in an affected area with bone chips, then allowing this coupling to heal so that the area fused becomes as one piece of bone.) Once this is accomplished the correction is maintained and the curve will not get worse.

Scoliosis can also occur from paralytic diseases such as polio, and when polio was prevalent, before the discovery of the anti-polio vaccines, fusions were occasionally carried out from the head to the sacrum—that is, the entire spine was made rigid.

Fusion seems like a drastic method of treatment, but scoliosis can produce terrible deformities in the back. Not only are they cosmetically disfiguring, they also produce compression of the chest cavity and hamper cardiac and pulmonary function. In addition, many scoliotic patients will suffer from severe back pain.

Intense efforts have been made recently to find the cause of scoliosis and to improve our methods of treatment. In fact several groups of international orthopaedic physicians devoted to research in this area have banded together to form the Scoliosis Society in order to pool their knowledge and research efforts.

As mentioned, scoliosis most frequently occurs in young girls. However, it also can affect anyone who is a victim of muscle paralysis or weakness, of congenital anomalies of the bones, or of tumors and infections about the spine.

We see, then, that postural and curvature problems are very significant in the production of back pain. Indeed, posture probably comes before anything else as the primary cause of back disorders. You might say that posture is the be-all and end-all of conventional back pain. Be-all in the sense that it's at the root of just about all conventional back disorders. And end-all in the sense that, properly established and maintained, it can be the end of just about all conventional disorders.

I'm not going to remind you to stand up straight, or throw those shoulders back, or keep chest out-stomach in. I've given you the mechanics of good posture, so as I end this chapter all I have to say to you is: "Think Posture!"

9.

The
Slipped Disc

Although Shakespeare never did compose a sonnet about back pain, he did write in one of his plays, *Timon of Athens*, these lines: "Thou cold sciatica, cripple our Senators that their limbs may halt as lamely as their manners." This was in 1608. Shakespeare obviously had knowledge—perhaps first-hand—of the painful and disabling effects of the back disorder that was universally known as *sciatica*.

Sciatica and Lumbago

Sciatica is severe pain in the lower back which often radiates down one or both legs and into the feet due to irritation of the sciatic nerve. Lumbago is severe pain in the lower back often accompanied by "locking" sensations and acute muscle spasm.

The terms *sciatica* and *lumbago* have been used for centuries to describe back pain. Until only relatively recently they were considered diseases in their own right rather than symptoms of something else altogether. Sciatica was not described in detail in a medical treatise until 1764. Then, in 1864, sciatica and lumbago were linked together for the first time. But not until 1933 was it shown conclusively that there was a single cause for the majority of cases of sciatica and lumbago. The cause was damaged lumbar intervertebral disc, or "slipped disc."

The discs were first described as long ago as 1555 by an anatomist called Vesalius. Three hundred years later a

German pathologist named Virchow described them in much greater detail, and remarked, in passing, about a tumor or swelling he had observed protruding into the spinal canal. A little over forty years later another German doctor, Ribbert, showed that these swellings were not really tumors but were irregularities produced by displacements of the intervertebral discs.

Such was the slow progress through the centuries toward solving the mystery of the major cause of sciatica and lumbago. Yet the final answer was still to come. A major advance was made in 1861 when Sicard, a French doctor, advanced the theory that sciatica was really due to irritation of some of the numerous nerve roots which join together in the lower back to form the sciatic nerve. Eleven years later an Italian doctor named Putti theorized that irritations of the sciatic nerve were due to intervertebral disc abnormalities.

The first true breakthrough from theory to fact did not come until 1933 when two American doctors, W. J. Mixter and J. C. Barr, reported on cases they had investigated at Massachusetts General Hospital. Their report described how intervertebral discs protrude and how such protrusion creates pressure on the roots of the sciatic and other nerves of the lower spinal canal, producing the symptoms of lumbago and sciatica.

The knowledge that sciatica was caused by pressure and irritation of the nerves was accepted by the medical profession only gradually. Indeed, several years would elapse and the world would become engulfed in the darkness of World War Two before this new theory found universal support.

By the end of the war, *Prolapsed Intervertebral Disc,* to give it the proper medical nomenclature, was acknowledged to be the principal cause not only of sciatica but of lumbago as well. (I must stress at this point that although it is the commonest cause of these two symptoms, *not all cases* of sciatica and lumbago are due to disc trouble.)

Although hindsight makes us wonder what took the medical profession so long to come to what now seems like an obvious conclusion, the concept of the Prolapsed Intervertebral Disc was a remarkable advance. At last it was possible to find one explanation to account for a wide variety of pains.

What Is a Disc?

I have heard people ask, "What did we do before they invented the slipped disc?" The answer is that the symptoms caused by slipped disc were always there, but because the reasons for them were unknown, the wrong label was put on the ailment. In effect, the symptoms were the disease.

Slipped disc is a disorder which has always existed. Nevertheless, it may be more common today than it was in past centuries due to the changed conditions of modern life which make us more prone to develop the disorder. There is little doubt—and I put a lot of credence in this notion—that our lack of physical exercise, plus our almost universally poor posture, makes our muscles slack and puts more pressure on our discs than they were designed to bear. Coupled with these factors is the type of work most of us do—our sedentary occupations—along with the soft beds we sleep on (remember, roughly one-third of our entire life is spent in bed). It's likely also that the anxieties and stresses created by modern life play a role in producing the condition.

The intervertebral disc is a circular capsule which fills the space between each of the vertebrae and is composed of three principal elements. The top and bottom of each disc consist of oval-shaped plates of gristle-like cartilage which conform to the shape of the bodies of the vertebrae and are integrally connected to them through the blending of their fibers with the fibers of the bodies. The second element is the tough tissue which, attached to the top and bottom plates, forms the rounded sides of the capsule—strips of elastic ligament overlaid obliquely and radially on one another to a thickness of about one-eighth of an inch. This wall is called the *annulus fibrosus*, and its elasticity allows the disc capsule to alter its shape in response to forces placed upon it, then rebound to its normal shape. Inside this capsule is the third element of the disc—the *nucleus pulposus* —in other words, the pulpy core. This pulpy core is a white, glistening, gel-like substance which acts hydraulically to give the disc capsule its shock-absorber capability.

Although most laymen tend to think of the disc as being the entire capsule, medically speaking only the pulpy core is the disc. When you hear of a disc being removed by

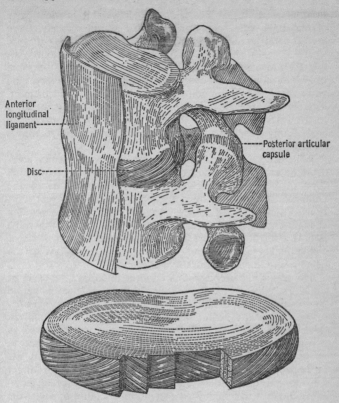

Anterior
longitudinal
ligament----

Disc----

----Posterior articular
capsule

*FIGS. 10 & 11 The intervertebral disc: above,
connecting two vertebrae; below, alone.*

surgery, it is only the core that is removed, not the capsule
itself.

One important function of the intervertebral discs is to
provide length and height to the spine. A man of average
height would only be four feet eight inches tall if he had
no discs, because the discs occupy 25 percent of the total
length of the spine.

Another function is to permit smooth, free, but controlled
movement between the vertebrae. The spine is capable of
supple movement in almost every direction. Flexion, exten-

sion, lateral tilting and rotation are all possible in most parts of the spine, yet except for the small articular facets, there are no solid bone-to-bone joints such as in the knee or hip. There are only the discs, and the discs, acting as joints, allow the movements of the spine to take place. At the same time they also limit movement. If they did not, every time you moved your spine you would find your back out of joint. That is why the cartilaginous plates are so firmly attached to the vertebrae and why the tough wall of the disc capsule is so firmly attached to the plates. This design allows movement within certain fixed limits.

With each movement of the spine the disc capsules compress or expand, depending on the nature of the motion. A forward bending, or flexion, for instance, will cause the front portions of the discs to compress and the rear portions to widen. All other motions create corresponding changes in the disc capsules' configuration. When the spine is held straight and there is no motion, the discs will be of equal thickness all around, except in certain regions of the spine where they are naturally wedge-shaped.

The shock-absorbing role is another important function of the discs. This protects the bones and keeps them intact to protect the spinal cord. The discs act as shock absorbers because their pulpy center behaves like an hydraulic fluid. In other words, the shape of the pulpy core can be altered as a result of sudden impact or compression, but it cannot be made to occupy a smaller space. At the moment and site of impact—whether through motion of the back or direct impact—the disc flattens out. Its tough elastic capsule, however, allows it to temporarily expand at the point opposite the point of impact so that the force is dissipated throughout the disc before it returns to its normal shape.

A disc is able to act as a shock absorber, then, because the pulp in its center is compressible. At the same time it has a definite volume, and no amount of pressure will reduce that volume. Although it will adopt any odd shape in response to an outside force, it cannot be expelled from its container. Under normal conditions, that is.

It is this pulpy core of the disc, which is liable to bulge against or squeeze out through a weak spot in the capsule's wall, that produces the abnormal condition known as slipped disc. This occurs when a portion of the *annulus*—the outside wall of the disc capsule—somehow degenerates and becomes soft, then either distends or ruptures. Once this hap-

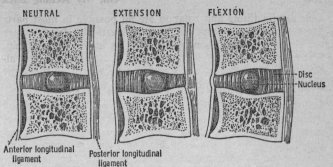

NEUTRAL   EXTENSION   FLEXION

Disc
Nucleus

Anterior longitudinal
ligament

Posterior longitudinal
ligament

FIG. 12 Views of spine in three situations—
neutral, extension and flexion—showing effect of
each on shape of disc.

pens, the damaged disc ceases to be effective both as an
intervertebral joint and as a shock absorber because the
pulpy interior is no longer properly contained in its space
within the walls of its capsule.

Discs are just as important in the spinal scheme of things
as the vertebrae they separate. They are not optional spare
parts that can be done without. While at first glance they
would not seem to be as strong as the very sturdy vertebral
bodies which they support and protect, they have to stand
up to the same stresses and strains. Since they are of softer
material you would think they would be more prone to injury, but this is not the case. Indeed, when a very great
force is applied to the spine it is often the bones which
break, not the discs.

Yet there is probably no other tissue in your body that
has to withstand such great forces so continuously as your
intervertebral discs. Therefore disc damage can and does
occur, usually in the form of the "slipped disc."

What Is a Slipped Disc?

As I've mentioned earlier, a slipped disc neither slips nor
is it, properly speaking, a disc. What we call a slipped disc
is really a complete breakdown of an intervertebral joint.

The first stage in this process usually occurs long before

the pulpy core of the disc is displaced—for that is what actually happens when we say a disc has slipped. The early stages generally pass unnoticed, for it is not until the displacement has actually taken place and the pulpy core has protruded onto adjacent areas of the spine that the typical symptoms appear.

The trouble usually starts gradually in the form of a degeneration and weakening at some spot on the side wall of the disc capsule—the annulus. The weakening generally occurs at the rear part of the capsule—the part closest to the spinal canal—most likely because the wall is thinner here than in the forward portions of the capsule. The degeneration takes the form of a softening of the tough elastic tissue in the wall which contains the pulp. Once the annulus is weakened the interior pressure of the pulp, coupled with a sudden force or twisting motion, might cause it to rupture, allowing part of the pulp to be squeezed out. This is called an "extruded disc." Or the annulus may just gradually stretch and bulge under the pressure of the pulp, like the weak spot in a balloon. Part of the pulp will fill the bulge and its pressure will gradually enlarge it, causing it to protrude. This is called a "protruded disc."

Once the annulus has either ruptured or merely bulged, a portion of the pulpy core of the disc capsule becomes displaced. The capsule will either partially or completely collapse, depending on the amount of pulp displaced, and the effect is like a partially or completely flat tire on your car. The cushioning function of the disc is lost, the balance of the spine is altered, and the muscles and ligaments surrounding the area become strained as they struggle to take up the load left by the collapsed disc.

But this is only the beginning. The protruding part of the capsule, or the extruded pulp if there has been a rupture in the annulus, will then bulge through the posterior longitudinal ligament that runs down the entire length of the spine between the discs and the spinal canal. The pressure of the pulp's displacement might even tear a hole in the ligament itself. At any rate, if the bulge is allowed to grow it will eventually press on the spinal cord or on nerve roots branching out from it, and severe pain will be the result.

The protrusion or extrusion of the nucleus pulposus is usually to one or the other side of the mid-line of the spinal canal. The result is that, as a rule, the symptoms of nerve pressure occur only on one side of the body.

This type of pressure causes irritation and inflammation of the nerves, which in turn provokes severe pain in the area supplied by the affected nerves. There are two separate manifestations of this irritation, but they usually occur together. The first is that the irritation of the sensory nerves produces a burning or searing pain in the area of the skin which normally sends messages along that nerve. The second is that pressure on the motor nerves causes the muscles supplied by them to go into states of uncontrolled contraction or spasm.

The uncontrollable spasms of the lower back muscles may be painful, but they are nature's way of helping the disorder to heal because they limit the movement of the spine and prevent more of the pulpy core from being displaced.

The disc does not slip back into place. The protrusion re-

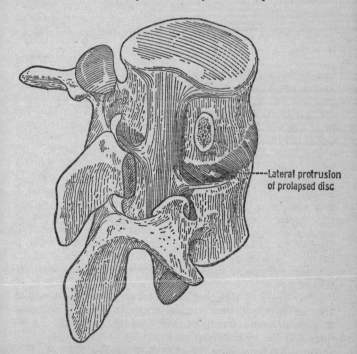

Lateral protrusion of prolapsed disc

FIG. 13   Typical disc protrusion.

mains and, if undisturbed, it heals in by scarring. However this remains a weak area and with further unprotected stress, greater protrusion is possible. When the pulp of the disc is actually extruded or squeezed through a rupture or hole in the annulus it lies against the nerve, causing considerable compression. This usually happens as an acute episode and results in severe pain with immediate neurological changes. If the extrusion is large enough, the compression may also involve the tail of the spinal cord and cause bladder and bowel disturbances. This situation constitutes a surgical emergency.

Several different kinds of pain may be produced by slipped disc, depending on the extent of displacement. In the first place there is a dull, aching pain which the victim finds difficult to locate. This is not a pain near the skin's surface which one could easily pinpoint. Rather, it is a deep dull ache in the spine and is probably seated in the affected disc itself or in the stretched ligament. It is not aggravated by all motions of the back, but bending movements will inflame it.

Although the pain due to pressure on the nerve root is usually felt in one or both legs in the form of sciatica due to the involvement of the sciatic nerve, it is also occasionally referred to the skin of the back or to one side above the hip joint. This pain is felt near the skin's surface, but once again it is hard to isolate because it's a referred pain and is not really on the surface at all.

The third type of pain is lumbago—a severe, sudden pain which causes the back to seize up. It is as if the muscles of the lumbar region have been suddenly gripped tight in a vise. If this pain comes on with dramatic suddenness it may disappear equally quickly. In some instances it will only appear for a few minutes, or a few hours, then just as quickly disappear. While it is present the victim's back is completely locked, permitting no movement. The pain is bearable as long as the back is kept perfectly still, but the slightest movement causes it to return with redoubled intensity.

After years of recurrent disc-associated back pain, a new type of backache may gradually emerge. This is the pain that occurs with inactivity, the kind in which the victim finds that his back stiffens up unless he keeps it supple with constant motion. It is characteristic of this type of pain that it is always worse after the back has been at rest, and mornings are usually the worst time. This pain is a symptom of arthritis, which can develop from long-term recurrent disc trouble that is allowed to progress.

Treatment of Slipped Disc

Setting aside for the moment slipped discs that are caused by direct accident, we've seen that the condition is ordinarily a progressive one. It appears first as a mild, aching discomfort in the lower back. At this point most sufferers tend to ignore it—classifying it as just another twinge and perhaps settling for a bit of liniment or an easy chair.

Let's say you are the person I'm describing. There may even be a realization that the little job of snow shoveling or rug vacuuming you just completed may have had something to do with it, but what's actually happened has been the beginning of the end. A few small fibers of a disc's annulus fibrosis have been stretched or pulled beyond their capacity, perhaps aided by the progressive weakening of tissue that's been building up over the years.

A few days or maybe a week later, let's say, you're putting out the trash or lifting a bundle of wet laundry. This time the pain comes a little quicker and stronger, because those annulus fibers, not yet fully recovered from the last episode, are even weaker.

Things can go along like this for months, years even, getting progressively worse and lasting a little longer each time until, finally, one day you do something that really knocks your back for a loop. That something can be as simple and ordinary as a sneeze or a cough. This time neither liniment nor an easy chair does any good. The pain you experience is giant-sized. It's not economy-sized, though, because by now it's going to cost you time and money.

Starting with those few weak and stretched annulus fibers that started to break down way back when, one of your discs has collapsed, perhaps even ruptured. The pulpy core may already have started to squeeze through the rupture, and everybody involved is in for a very hard time.

Especially you!

As the star of this unhappy and painful drama you, the patient, will find yourself in bed, usually lying on one side with your legs pulled up to your chest to relieve the pressure on the nerve. The tired, weary muscles of your back, constantly straining to find some position of comfort, will begin to ache of their own account from the effort.

If the damage to your disc is the result of an accident of some kind, there is at least a small advantage—you'll probably get immediate attention and treatment, without waiting, without trying to kid yourself that it's really not all that serious. You will thus get started on the long job of getting well that much sooner.

No matter the cause, once a diagnosis has been made that one of your discs has begun to protrude, the first phase of treatment must be complete bed rest in order to relieve all strain on the area and give the disc a chance to stabilize and heal. If you were to continue to stand on your feet, the weight of your body would compress the affected disc and cause additional protrusion. This would sooner or later lead to complete rupture of the annulus, if it hadn't already happened.

By complete bed rest I mean *complete bed rest*. That means no sitting up to take meals, no getting up to use the bathroom or to take a shower because you can't stand yourself another moment. If this is impossible to achieve at home, then you should undergo it in a hospital. It is true that some patients with disc damage manage to break the rules without serious consequences. However, you don't want to take chances with your back, and the most you have to lose is a little time in exchange for giving the damaged disc a chance to heal.

If you were my patient I would definitely suggest hospitalization in any case of disc protrusion. Since lying on your back with your legs straight out is not the best form of rest treatment for protruded discs, I would arrange to use a routine pelvic traction device. If you've heard about traction you are likely to have an image of some torturous medieval device which stretches your spine and causes all sorts of additional agonies. Your fears would be unfounded. The type of traction I would employ is a simple device consisting of a girdle-like belt which wraps around your waist and hips. Straps are attached to the sides and each strap is in turn attached to weights which hang over the foot of the bed. I use approximately ten pounds of weight for each strap, lowering or raising the amount of weight depending on the size of the patient.

The traction is *not* intended to stretch or pull your vertebrae apart in order to allow the disc to slip back into place, as many people believe. The disc will not slip back. The purpose of the traction is to raise your pelvis and reduce the curve in your lumbar spine, thereby relieving the pressure of the protruded disc on your nerves and relieving muscle spasm. Sorry to deflate the myth about traction—it is only an aid to treatment, not treatment itself.

Along with traction I would give you pain medication and muscle relaxants. Hot packs applied to the affected region are sometimes helpful, but their use is really limited. X-rays and blood tests would be done, and I would be able to examine you daily and evaluate your progress. If no evidence of nerve root damage existed, I would then concern myself with reducing your muscle spasm. If there were neurological changes, these would have to be watched very carefully.

After about ten or twelve days of this type of bed rest, with good progress on your part—absence of spasms, return of sensation and motor power, and obvious improvement in your general comfort—I would then start to gradually put you on your feet. Initially you would be allowed out of bed twice a day for ten minutes. If you tolerated this well, I would slowly increase your duration of standing and walking. But I would permit no immediate sitting down, except for the bathroom. You would simultaneously begin gentle exercises in bed. Over the next seven or eight days you should progress to the point where you can be up for an hour without discomfort—the minimum requirement for discharge and going home. In order to function at home, even on a minimal level, you must be able to tolerate being out of bed for one hour. Sitting is always the most strenuous activity for your back except for bending and lifting, and so I would have you delay doing any sitting for a long time.

Once home you would continue daily to increase your activities and add specific exercises to your regimen. When you were able to be up and about most of the day (this takes about two or three weeks), you could consider returning to work on a part-time basis if your work was not strenuous and if it did not require much traveling.

It now becomes clear that a real slipped disc, treated without an operation, requires about six to eight weeks in order to heal sufficiently to enable you to return to even part-time normal activities. Is that a big sigh, I hear? Well, the best treatment is to prevent the entire problem, which only you can do. I have described the general conservative post-diagnosis treatment. Of course, there are exceptions. Some people are better in one week, while others may require six weeks of bed rest and traction. Notice, I have not prescribed a single back brace.

What happens if you don't get better? The spasms continue, the neurological changes persist or even get worse—what then? Since I have been seeing you every day, I am well aware that you are not improving. At the end of a week with no improvement, I would obtain a myelogram. (In the presence of serious neurological deficits, I would have had a myelogram done immediately when you were admitted.) If the myelogram confirms the presence of large disc protrusion, I would then feel it necessary to proceed with surgery and remove the disc. But if the myelogram does not reveal a herniation of the disc or if the defect is very slight, I would then continue with bed rest and traction for an additional period of time.

Each disc patient I treat has his particular make-up, and everyone's degree of disc damage differs from everyone else's. This makes it very difficult to predict the outcome of a disc problem, but I can say in general that of one hundred disc patients I see in my office, thirty of them will require hospitalization. Of these thirty patients, fifteen will need an operation. Before I describe disc operations and their results, two examples of the difficulty of diagnosis and prediction might be illuminating.

A middle-aged man, dynamic, successful, chairman of the board of a billion-dollar-a-year company, was brought to my office in excruciating pain. He was tilted to one side and his back spasms were so severe he could hardly talk. He was in too much pain for a thorough examination, but I was able to determine that his neurological status was intact. I had him immediately admitted to the hospital and placed on bed rest with pelvic traction. He was given adequate pain relievers and muscle relaxants. His X-rays were normal. After three days, he was out of bed and walking. He had no pain, and returned to work the next day.

Remarkable? Yes, but he had severe lumbo-sacral spasm, probably associated with fatigue, poor posture, and excessive sitting. His attack had occurred while he was at a board meeting. His pencil had dropped to the floor and he leaned over sideways to pick it up. He felt a sudden contraction in his back and was unable to move. When giving his history he told me that the pain was radiating into his leg, but upon further questioning I learned that the pain went down his thigh only to his knee, not below. Classical sciatic pain radiates all the way down the leg to the foot. Depending upon the nerve root involved, the pain may localize near the heel or near the big toe. So, then, this gentleman did not have a genuine disc protrusion and he recovered in a short time. However, I started him on an exercise program because he now had a definite lumbo-sacral weakness. The next time he strains his lower back his disc may not hold up and could extrude—that is, slip. So a preventive program is necessary to strengthen his back to reduce the possibility of another strain.

Another patient, a forty-two-year-old, overweight female who was employed as a legal secretary, had been having bouts of back pain with radiation down her right leg to the foot for several years. She had been hospitalized twice, each time for three weeks. She had worn different types of braces almost continuously. She had had diathermy, injections, hot packs, even chiropractic manipulation. She told me that she had recently been seen by another orthopaedist who had recommended surgery. She was absolutely terrified of surgery and would go to any length in order to avoid it.

Well, my examination revealed that she had moderate muscle spasm of her back, some atrophy of her right leg muscles with concurrent weakness, loss of ankle reflexes and decreased sensation in her foot. I told her that in view of her history and finding she probably would require surgery, but that it would be worthwhile to first try extensive bed rest and traction. We tried for six weeks. At the end of the third week she was no better. She still had pain and her neurological findings were unchanged.

A myelogram revealed a large bulging disc between the 5th lumbar vertebra and the sacrum. She still refused surgery. At the end of six weeks of complete bed rest without even bathroom privileges, she showed improvement. The pain was just about absent. Her straight-leg raising and other signs were improved, and her muscle tone was better. But sensation was still decreased. In another three weeks she was at home, on her exercise program. Eight weeks after her discharge she was back to work part-time, and at the end of sixteen weeks she was working full-time.

Now, she has not been cured. She still gets occasional back and leg pain and must rest at home for a few days. The numbness in her foot persists and she continues to have a limp. However, she is happy. She did not want an operation. She can work, and she tolerates her limitations in rather good spirits.

The moral of this story is that we treat the patient, not necessarily the disc. Contrary to much popular belief, most surgeons do not sit in their offices with scalpels in hand just waiting for disc cases to show up. We would much rather save a disc than excise it, if that's at all possible and practicable. Whether we can or not often depends on the patient—whether he or she is willing to go through the long, quiescent period of treatment in bed.

Surgical Treatment

The decision as to whether or not to operate is not difficult. In some instances the patient is so fed up with his pain, weakness and disability that he practically begs for surgery. At other times the doctor must make the suggestion and explain the reasons for it. No one particularly enjoys undergoing surgery, yet there are times when this is the only sensible treatment.

Surgery would be called for in your case if you were to have persistent pain and it was not relieved by traction and bed rest, or if you were to have pronounced weakness and numbness of the leg and the neurological deterioration was progressive.

What does the surgeon do? I'll spare you the gory details, but in essence he begins by cleaning off the rear portion of the vertebral arch at the site of the damaged disc, removing the *ligamenta flava* and part of the *lamina* of the vertebra, and exposing the *dura* of the spinal cord, at the same time isolating the affected nerve roots. He then locates the disc herniation, either visually or by feel. He removes the extruded portion of the damaged disc and then, with special instruments, extracts the remainder of the disc's pulp from the collapsed capsule.

"My goodness," patients often exclaim, "what happens to the empty space?" Not very much happens to the space. It is already very thin due to the collapse of the disc. After the disc is removed the space gradually fills in with scar tissue. Obviously the scar tissue does not replace the function of the nucleus pulposus—it is not an efficient shock absorber—but it will fill up the space. Over a long period of time the space between the two vertebrae may also be bridged by bone tissue which grows between the vertebrae, creating a kind of spontaneous fusion which adds stability to the area.

I would emphasize here that treatment does not end with the removal of a damaged disc. The slipped disc, although a genuine disorder in itself, is also a symptom of a more insidious disorder—instability and weakness of the back in general. Removing the disc does not strengthen the back and erase its general instability. To achieve that takes, first, the healing process, and then a gradual building up of the back once the patient has recovered from the effects of the surgery.

The success of a disc operation is dependent upon three things: competent surgery, good post-operative care, and faithful post-operative back therapy. The surgeon is responsible for the quality of the first two. You are responsible for carrying out the third part. Although I have never officially tabulated the results of my slipped disc operations, I would estimate that 85 percent of the patients I have operated on for this condition were able to resume their normal physical activities (I exclude strenuous sports like football).

Fusion

You might be wondering by now about this business called fusion. Certainly if you've been involved with disc problems you've heard about it. Many orthopaedic and neurosurgeons routinely fuse every intervertebral space from which a disc has been removed. Others believe that fusion is rarely necessary. Thus there is a dichotomy of opinion. I believe the answer lies somewhere in between the extremes.

You'll recall that fusion is a procedure a surgeon uses to connect the vertebral bodies in order to immobilize and stabilize the spine in the region of the removed disc. He does this by bringing in strips of bone from outside the region—usually from the pelvis—and grafting them to the vertebral bones.

If you have had a long history of chronic back pain and instability associated with your disc, I would then advise fusion along with disc removal in order to stabilize that region of your spine which has been compromised and has been generally resistant to clinical treatment and therapy. And if your X-rays revealed bone abnormalities such as *spina bifida* or *asymmetric facets* associated with your disc collapse, I would also recommend fusion because these factors are most likely the cause of your problem.

If, on the other hand, your symptoms were of more recent onset, and you had little prior history of chronic back disability, I would then recommend only excising the disc and omitting fusion. Fusion certainly has its advantages, and is even necessary in certain types of disc disorders, but it requires a considerably long post-operative healing period.

All post-operative recuperation requires extended bed rest, just as in non-surgical treatment. Once the damaged site has healed, it is important that an exercise program be undertaken for the purpose of strengthening the back and avoiding future pain and disc problems.

The Cervical Discs

The problems I have discussed so far in this chapter have pertained mostly to the discs of the lower back—the lumbar discs. However, degeneration of the cervical discs, the ones that run along the neck portion of your spine, is not an uncommon phenomenon. This is often associated with arthritic changes in the neck as well, so that there develops a combination of bony spurs plus disc protrusion which creates pressure on the spinal cord and nerve roots.

When the cervical discs are involved the symptoms are confined to the upper extremities. They usually consist of pain centered in the neck and radiating down through the shoulders and arms to the hands. If the nerve compression is excessive, the victim will develop weakness and atrophy of the forearm and hand muscles and loss of sensation in the fingers and hand.

Basically the same course of events which I have described for the lumbar region of the spine is followed in the cervical region, but there are a few significant differences between the two. One is that the neck is not subjected to the same stresses, loads and forces that the lumbar spine is subjected to, so that cervical disc protrusions are not very large. Another is that the portion of the spinal cord that lies within the cervical region of the spinal canal is much larger and contains many more nerves. Consequently, in some respects damage to this area can be much more serious than to the lumbar region because it involves the entire spinal cord. Except for those patients who have sudden injuries to their necks, such as cervical sprain ("whiplash" injury is the term beloved by lawyers but abhorred by all orthopaedists) or a specific trauma which may lead to early or premature degeneration of a cervical disc, cervical disc problems are more common to older people than younger.

The treatment program is similar to that of lower disc-caused back pain: bed rest and cervical traction in more severe cases, cervical collars in milder cases. Occasionally surgery is required to remove a really recalcitrant disc, and in these cases fusion is routinely performed.

Ultimately all weak backs develop disc degeneration or herniation. If you have already been through disc treatment, you'll know how important exercise therapy is for avoiding recurrence. If you've not yet been through disc treatment, but do have the kind of weak, unstable back and chronic attacks of pain and spasm I've been describing, you can be sure you're on your way to serious disc trouble. The one chance you have of cutting it off before the condition progresses to that point is to go to work on your back—through improved posture and exercise therapy.

10.

Congenital and Developmental Defects

The vast bulk of all backache is avoidable. In the main, there are only two simple considerations you have to be aware of to avoid back pain. One is how you handle yourself when making an extra or unusual physical effort, particularly lifting. The other is keeping your back in condition through proper posture and use. If you don't get to use your back much, then you should make up for its inactivity with exercise. As the old saying goes, the blacksmith's arm is strong because he uses it.

Except for a few conditions like infections, tumors, severe accidental injuries, and uncontrollable developmental defects, all of the backache limping around today could probably have been avoided by observance of a few easily understood and not inconvenient precautions.

Nevertheless these conditions over which we have no control *do* exist, and it's time now to have a brief look at a few of the more common ones.

Two groups of spinal defects exist: the congenital group, in which the particular defect or anomaly is present at birth; and the developmental group, in which the defect is not present at birth but develops after birth. We've already seen two examples of this group—scoliosis and Scheuermann's Disease.

Congenital Defects

The miracle of conception and birth—the union of sperm and ovum to form a single cell which then divides and re-divides until a recognizable fetus is formed and continues to develop—never ceases to amaze me. That this extraordinarily complicated process almost always culminates without error is an even greater source of wonderment.

Yet errors do occasionally occur, and when they take the form of spinal defects we must recognize them as early as possible and remedy them as best we can within the limits of our medical knowledge and experience.

The most frequent of the relatively rare spinal defects that do occur come under the name *spina bifida*. Spina bifida is the failure of part of the spine—the posterior neural arch or the rear portion of one or more of the vertebrae —to develop. In the embryonic state the rear portions of the vertebra are the last to form. In a certain amount of cases this part of the spine fails to form at all. Thus the spinal cord has nothing to hold it in. As a result the cord, with its coverings (*meninges*), forms a sac which protrudes through the skin of the back.

This abnormality may affect only a short portion of the spine or it may affect a lengthy portion. When it is a large abnormality it will compromise the function of the nerves and cause paralysis and lack of sensation in the lower extremities, as well as bladder and bowel paralysis. This condition, called *meningomyelocele*, requires special long-term medical care.

When it's a small defect, however, the spinal cord is not likely to be compromised in any significant way. Nevertheless the absence of enclosing bone at the rear of a vertebra, which is what spina bifida refers to, can impair the structural stability of the involved spinal segment and lead to pain. The segments most frequently involved are those at the junction of the lumbar and sacral portions of the spine.

The condition is difficult to diagnose before a child is five or six years old, because the defect will not show up on X-ray until that general age. A clinical sign of the small defect is the appearance of a small dimple at the bottom of the spine with a tuft of hair growing over it. The big defect is obvious.

From statistics gathered during World War Two it was learned that approximately 20 percent of all Army inductees had this defect in one degree or another, mostly minor. In most instances a spina bifida defect is not productive of pain or disability. However, when a patient does have continuing severe back pain and I observe the presence of the defect on X-rays, he might require surgical fusion to correct the condition.

Another general type of congenital defect is found in the lumbar region of the spine. A child may be born with only four lumbar vertebrae. Or, on the other hand, he may be born with six, instead of the normal five. Or one or more of the vertebral bodies may be incompletely formed, resulting in what are known as *hemivertebrae*. In other instances two or more vertebrae will fail to separate from one another, causing congenital fusion. Still another defect occurs when the *articular facets* of one or more vertebrae do not form evenly but instead are asymmetric, causing irregular motion in the vertebral joints. Although all of these congenital anomalies are relatively uncommon, they can all cause back pain. When the pain is severe and recurring, surgery may be the only corrective treatment.

Abnormality in the number of lumbar vertebrae is not as significant a defect as partially formed vertebrae (hemivertebrae) or congenitally fused vertebrae. If only four lumbar vertebrae are present, we say that there is *sacralization* of the 5th lumbar vertebra—that is, the normal 5th lumbar vertebra has been incorporated into the sacrum. On the other hand, if we count six lumbar vertebrae, we then say that there is *lumbarization* of the first sacral segment —that is, the upper part of the sacrum is separated from the main body of the sacrum and appears as an additional lumbar vertebra. Either of these conditions can produce pain and instability, but they are normally responsive to careful management of the back.

Hemivertebrae and congenitally fused vertebrae usually result in another form of scoliosis—called congenital scoliosis. This type differs from the scoliosis I described in the chapter on posture and curvature because it occurs with equal frequency in men and, although the treatment procedures are the same, is less susceptible to surgical correction.

The defect of asymmetric articular facets falls more or less into the same category as an abnormal number of vertebrae as far as instability and pain are concerned. Although they can cause both, they can be managed without too much difficulty. Actually, all of these anomalies were once thought to be much more significant as causes of back pain prior to the discovery and understanding of the role of the "slipped disc." Since then it has become obvious that these defects play only a minor role in causing back pain and disability.

Developmental Defects

Aside from excessive lumbar lordosis (swayback), excessive dorsal kyphosis (hump back) and scoliosis (lateral curvature), which I've discussed in Chapter 8, there are two other major developmental defects with long, complicated names which often go hand in glove to produce acute back pain and instability.

These are *spondylolysis* and—are you ready?—*spondylolisthesis*. Of all the devilish exhibits in the back's chamber of horrors, these two abnormalities are every bit as nefarious and shifty as could be expected of things with names like those. The first of these—spondylolysis—is nefarious because it is a condition in which a portion of bone connecting the upper and lower articular facets of a vertebra is missing. The second—spondylolisthesis—is shifty because it is a condition which, due to the lack of bone, produces a slipping of the spine at the defective site.

For our purposes we can gather both of these confusing names under one word—*spondy*. This is how it works. Early in the growth of the spine there develops a loss of continuity of bone in a vertebra—that piece of bone which connects the superior and inferior articular facets. In its effect it is much like a fracture—a gap grows between the two elements. The gap becomes filled with fibrous and cartilaginous tissue. This is the first of the spondys.

Then, because these tissues are soft and not rigid, as normal bone is, they allow abnormal motion or slipping to occur between the bones. This is the second of the two spondys. The first spondy, then, is the defect itself; the second is the result of the defect—the slipping forward of one vertebra on another.

What causes spondy? For many years it was felt to be a congenital defect and that the portion of vertebral bone was missing at birth. In almost all instances the defect occurs between the lowest lumbar vertebra and the sacrum. Studies of newborns' spines, however, failed to reveal this defect, so it became apparent that the defect was not congenital. Once that was established, the next line of reasoning was that it resulted from some sort of chronic childhood strain.

At the present time it is generally accepted that spondy is caused by chronic strain on the 5th lumbar vertebra, with excessive lumbar lordosis playing a significant role in the production of the strain. Since excessive lordosis is greatest at the lumbo-sacral junction, it is the 5th lumbar vertebra that is most frequently involved.

The presence of either of these forms of spondy can cause lower back pain, and in the case of slippage, radiation of the pain into the legs through the effect of the slippage on the sciatic nerve. The simple fact is that if you have the first form of spondy, you probably will sooner or later develop the second form.

Sometimes the trouble will not show up until the late teens. It appears with increasing frequency in the adult years as the burdens of living, both literally and figuratively, come to bear. No one with spondy can hope to sneak through the years of maturity and old age without distress unless he is extraordinarily lucky. Sooner or later the maverick front portion of that all-important 5th lumbar vertebra begins to creep forward, slipping across the platform provided for it by the sacrum below and carrying with it the whole spinal assembly above along a path of ever-increasing distortion and displacement. The intervening disc, designed to serve other needs, is inexorably stretched and weakened by the shifting vertebra. Nearby nerve lines, caught in the increasingly abnormal conditions created over the years, become inflamed and irritated.

This is spondylolisthesis. As a matter of hard, unpalatable fact, although it doesn't always get worse, there is no way of correcting this insidious condition once it has started —that is, there is no way the spine can be brought back to its proper alignment and held there. Surgery can arrest it, however, through fusion. The operation consists of fusing the 5th lumbar vertebra to the sacrum. Frequently the 4th lumbar vertebra will be included in the fusion in order to make certain that the area is stable and no further slippage of the 5th vertebra occurs. Once this is done and the area has healed, exercise therapy and careful management of the back are necessary in order to prevent further pain and disability.

In older people a different kind of spondylolisthesis exists, but I shall save discussion of that for a later chapter.

11.

Infections and Tumors

Infections and tumors of the spine are now relatively rare disorders, but since we're touching all the bases in this book we must have a short consideration of them as causes of back pain.

Before the era of antibiotics and antitubercular drugs, infections of the spine occurred all too frequently and produced prolonged pain and disability. The only kind of treatment which seemed effective was spinal fusion, the area fused being the particular region of the spine damaged by the infection. Such fusions took a long, long time to heal and patients would be required to lay abed for many months. Besides which, the results were not always good.

Tuberculosis of the spine was the most common type of backbone infection. The infection was so common that it was given the name of the man who first described it in 1779, Sir Percivall Pott. *Pott's Disease* was a worldwide disorder, yet it was only one of a number of types of tuberculosis that infected the spine.

The incidence of both general infections of the vertebral bones (osteomyelitis of the vertebrae, or *spondylitis*) and specific tubercular infections of the spine has been dramatically reduced since the discovery of antibiotics and antitubercular drugs (some of which, like *Streptomycin*, are antibiotics). I still encounter a few of these infections each year, however, and they are certainly worth a place in any discussion on back pain and its causes.

Spondylitis

Osteomyelitis of the spine, or spondylitis, is caused by bacterial infection, usually by a *staphylococcus* organism. Even rarer type organisms can infect the spine, including fungus, but staph is the most common cause of infection.

Infection may occur in one of two ways—*hematogenously*, which is to say that the bacteria are carried by the blood, or through *direct implantation* of the bacteria. Hematogenous infection is the most frequent type.

It works this way. Bacteria get into the bloodstream and are carried to the vertebral bodies in the spine. Within the bodies of the infected vertebrae the blood "pools," or forms microscopic swamps. In these stagnant media, the virulent bacterial organisms begin to grow and overcome the natural body defenses. From that moment on, the infection begins.

The infection usually starts in a single vertebra and then spreads to an adjoining one by breaking through the bone tissue and eating into the protective ligaments above and below. Meanwhile the victim becomes aware of general back pain, usually in the lumbar region, and begins to experience fever. As the infection progresses the victim feels sick and suffers acute loss of appetite. Many diagnoses can be confused by this clinical picture—the disease might be mistaken for kidney stones, kidney infections, pneumonia, even the flu.

The proper diagnosis is established by eliminating the other possible causes through routine lab tests, and by properly evaluating the nature and site of tenderness and muscle spasm. X-ray indications of the infection will usually not appear for the first ten to fourteen days, so in the early stages X-rays are not conclusive.

Once the infection has been diagnosed and X-rays are able to show which vertebrae are involved, it is important to establish the type and nature of the infecting organism. This information is obtained by doing a *needle biopsy*— extracting a portion of the infecting material from the site of the infection with a needle and syringe.

The thought of this procedure may be frightening, but in actuality it is carefully controlled and does not cause any great discomfort. An *image intensifier*, which is a machine similar to a fluoroscope and which gives the doctor direct

vision into the bone, is commonly used for accurate place-
ment of the needle, and whatever pain might be involved
is shut off by injection of a local anaesthetic.

Once the infecting material is drawn out it is immediately
sent to the lab for culture studies and for determination of
type. General antibiotics are started, and when the infecting organism is identified in the lab the specific antibiotics
to which it is most susceptible are then administered to the
patient.

The earlier any spinal infection is diagnosed, the better
the prognosis will be and the less destruction of bone
will occur. If bone destruction is advanced—and by that
I mean loss of bone substance and support—then surgery
will be necessary in order to repair the damage. This consists of scraping out the remaining infection and then fusing
the affected parts of the spine. All these things mean a long
period of disability, and are all the more reason why you
should get an early diagnosis of any back pain you have.

Tuberculosis

Tuberculosis, too, is an infection of the spine and is an
even more insidious disease then spondylitis. The tubercular
organisms are carried to the vertebral bodies by the bloodstream. Their growth rate is slow, so there is not a sudden
or acute onset of symptoms. As the tubercles grow, the
bone is slowly destroyed and abscesses develop as adjacent
vertebrae become involved. The abscesses and scar tissue
that grow in reaction to the disease will often encroach upon
the spinal canal and cause compression or pinching of the
spinal cord, resulting in partial or total paralysis of the lower
body. Indeed, before adequate treatment for tuberculosis
(Pott's Disease) was developed, roughly 20 percent of spinal
tuberculosis victims developed lower-limb paralysis.

The abscesses formed by the infection slowly enlarge and
spread into muscle layers. Tubercular abscesses are capable
of traveling very great distances in the body, so that an infection in the upper spine may eventually drain from the
groin.

Early symptoms are few: mild pain, low-grade fever, loss
of appetite, night sweats—all symptoms that can be confused
with a host of other problems. The symptoms persist and
gradually become more severe. Physical examination won't

show much except for local tenderness at the infection site
and a limitation of motion, signs common to various other
disorders. A chest X-ray will most likely show no active TB
unless the chest contains an old, quiescent area of infection.
X-rays of the spine will not show much unless the disease
is in its more advanced stages. Usually the dorsal spine is
most frequently attacked by tuberculosis, but any part of
the spine is vulnerable.

Specific skin tests for tuberculosis are helpful in diagnosis,
but its presence can only be positively confirmed by needle
biopsy, as in the case of spondylitis. If the diagnosis is able
to be made before the disease has led to the collapse of the
vertebral bodies and before abscess formation is too far
along, the patient may be treated with bed rest and antitubercular drugs.

But when bone destruction and large abscess formation
has occurred, surgery is the only corrective treatment. This
consists of exposing the vertebral bodies, removing the abscesses and the infected portion of the spine, then replacing
the bone removed with bone-graft struts in order to prevent
vertebra collapse. Fusion completes the operative procedure
and prognosis, after sufficient healing time, is generally fa-
vorable.

A very interesting fact with regard to tuberculosis and other spinal infections is that the intervertebral disc is generally
spared from the disease because it has essentially no blood
supply. Tubercular bacteria need blood and oxygen to survive, as do most infecting organisms.

Meningitis

Infections of the spinal column are called spondylitis. Infections of the spinal cord are called meningitis, and these
are very serious indeed. Meningitis can be produced by bacteria or, more rarely, by a virus. No matter what the infecting organism is, the symptoms are always similar and
severe—spasms, pain, rigidity of the neck. When the infection is caused by the very virulent *meningococcus* bacteria,
the victim will likely have very high fever as well.

Meningitis is not usually confused with more routine back
problems when it comes time for a diagnosis—the symptoms are clear and unmistakable. Nevertheless, in the early
stages of a viral infection causing meningitis, the patient's

symptoms may be simply nothing more than back pain. It is therefore important, whenever a patient does complain of back pain, that the doctor test his reflexes in order to determine whether meningitis is present or not. Hyperactive reflexes in the presence of back pain and high fever are a sure sign of meningitis.

It is *always* desirable to diagnose meningitis in its early stages, before it has a chance to progress too far. It is treatable and curable with penicillin and other antibiotic drugs, but if it is allowed to progress, serious neurological complications can result.

Closely associated with spinal meningitis is *poliomyelitis*. We can all be grateful to the discoverers of the anti-polio vaccines. They have made this dread paralytic disease of the spinal cord almost obsolete.

Benign Tumors

Tumors of the spine can be divided into two groups: benign and malignant. Benign tumors are those that do not spread throughout the body and which can be removed or treated locally. Malignant tumors are those that do spread. They can involve the spine primarily, which is to say they grow somewhere in the spinal column and then spread to other parts of the body, or they can involve it secondarily, that is, grow elsewhere and spread to the spine.

Benign tumors of the bone are uncommon. They may consist of an abnormal bone growth which is limited to a vertebra's pedicle, in which case they are responsible for what is known as *osteoblastoma*. Or they may be small inflammatory lesions which produce the entity called *osteoid osteoma* in younger individuals. Or they may constitute a partial replacement of a vertebral body by a network of blood vessels—this is called *hemangioma* and, when it occurs, which is seldom, it may produce no symptoms at all.

The important thing about all these growths is that they be recognized for what they are—benign tumors—and treated accordingly. Local excision of the osteoblastoma and osteoid osteoma is usually all that's required to relieve whatever painful symptoms exist. A hemangioma of the bone requires no treatment at all unless it is so extensive that the vertebral body collapses. Then, corrective fusion surgery is employed.

Other benign tumors may involve the back without arising in the bones. One of the commonest soft-tissue tumors is *neurofibroma*. Relatively rare, these tumors form lumps anywhere from pea-size to grapefruit-size. They can appear anywhere in the body, including on the skin. Often large brownish discolorations are noted on the skin (café-au-lait spots) in conjunction with these masses. The lumps themselves consist of fibrous nerve tissue and are most often found on or about nerves. Their presence in the neural canal or on the spinal cord can cause quite a bit of pain. The symptoms mimic those of a herniated disc due to the pressure of the lump on the nerve roots. A myelogram is usually very helpful in enabling the diagnostician to distinguish between the two conditions. When a neurofibroma is removed, which is the usual treatment, the symptoms subside, but the lesion may repeat itself in other parts of the body.

Fatty tumors, or *lipomas,* in the subcutaneous tissue of the skin or between the muscle layers of the back often arise, but they are generally without any painful symptoms. Unless they do produce tenderness through enlargement, they need only be diagnosed, then ignored.

Malignant Primary Tumors

Malignant tumors of the spine are, fortunately, rare. However, cancer is not rare, and malignant tumors arising in other parts of the body can and frequently do spread to the spine. Indeed, symptoms of pain and discomfort in the spine or general area of the back are, not infrequently, the first signs of cancer in other parts of the body, especially those parts adjacent to or near the spine.

Primary cancers of the spine may arise, when they do arise, in any portion of the spine. They may be slow-growing and invade other tissues only by localized extensions, such as the *chordoma.* Or they may be rapid-growing and spread extensively, such as in the virulent and deadly disease known as *osteogenic sarcoma.* Another type of bone cancer is *multiple myeloma.* This tumor occurs as a result of an abnormal proliferation of bone-marrow cells and may appear in many different bones simultaneously. It is generally seen in people between the ages of forty to sixty and appears on X-ray as a "hole" in the bone. Although the tumor may be first seen in the spine, X-rays of other bones may reveal further areas of involvement.

The initial symptoms of these malignant tumors are pain, loss of appetite and weight loss. When X-rays reveal bone destruction and possible cancer it is then necessary to obtain an immediate biopsy—preferably *open biopsy* as opposed to needle biopsy—in order to secure an accurate diagnosis. Blood tests are also helpful, especially in the diagnosis of multiple myeloma.

Unfortunately, as in many other body cancers, once diagnosed, primary spinal cancer treatment is limited. If a chordoma is small, local excision may be attempted, but it will usually recur. Growth is slow, however, and a chordoma victim may survive many years.

Osteogenic sarcoma of the spine can only be treated by radiation, but this usually has little effect. Consequently the outlook for this disease is poor. Multiple myeloma also has a poor prognosis, but chemotherapy (the use of chemical cell-killing agents), combined with radiation treatment, often slows the growth of this cancer and relieves the pain.

Other even more uncommon primary spinal tumors exist, but I think the ones described are sufficient to give you an appreciation of the seriousness of these tumors.

Malignant Secondary Tumors

Metastatic tumors to the spine—secondary tumors, those which spread to the spine from other sources in the body—may occur with almost any cancer. The five most common sources of secondary spinal cancer are from the breast, thyroid, lung, prostate and kidney. It has been established by autopsy studies that people who die of cancer show evidence of *bone metastasis*—cancerous involvement of the bone, regardless of the original site of the cancer—in 85 percent of the cases. Certainly, then, when a patient complains of back pain and has what appears to be a destructive lesion of spinal bone on X-ray, the possibility of this lesion having been produced from another site must be strongly considered in diagnosis.

The X-ray appearances of a tumor of the spine and of an infection of the spine differ considerably. As I mentioned earlier, infections tend to involve contiguous or immediately adjacent vertebrae. Tumors, on the other hand, tend to de-

stroy or collapse one vertebral body and then skip a few
segments to attack another, either above or below. In addition, there is no infection-abscess shadow on the X-ray, but
occasionally the X-ray appearance is not distinctive enough
for differentiation.

The diagnosis of a metastatic cancer to the spine is determined by discovering the primary site, either with specific
tests such as *radioactive thyroid studies, intravenous pyelo-
grams* of the kidney, X-rays of the lung, or by biopsy of the
spinal lesion itself and determination of the primary site of
the cancer by identifying the type of abnormal tissue present
in the secondary site.

Treatment is first directed at the primary tumor. Then the
spinal manifestation is treated with radiation, hormones or
chemotherapy.

Malignant tumors are not confined to the skeleton or bones
of the back. They also arise in soft tissues. Lesions such as
fibrosarcoma and *liposarcoma* will occur in the muscle and
fatty layers of the back, while lesions such as malignant
schwannoma may occur about the spinal cord. These are so
rare that an elaboration of the tumors and their nature is
not necessary for our purposes here. If possible, they should
be surgically excised. When the tumor is completely removed
prognosis is good; otherwise they recur and spread.

This discussion of cancer in the back may strike you as a
bit disturbing or morbid, yet it is vitally necessary if you are
to have a complete understanding of your back, and an appreciation of back pain itself. It is my hope that such an appreciation will alert you to all the possibilities of back pain
and will prevent those few of you who might be in for a case
of back cancer, or any other kind of cancer, from allowing
such diseases to progress beyond the help of treatment.

A case in point is that of the fifty-six-year-old man who
was recently referred to me by his family doctor with a case
of "slipped disc." Although his preliminary signs on examination were suggestive of a disc problem, the myelogram I
ordered for him dispelled this suggestion. Yet he still had a lot
of pain in his back and the limited mobility common to a
lower back disorder. After a rectal examination and several
other tests, I discovered he had cancer of his prostate gland
and that the cancer had metastasized to his lumbar spine.
The metastasis was not visible on routine X-rays, but was
confirmed when I instituted special radioactive studies of his
spine. He had once had a disc problem, but this was now

dormant. Once his prostate tumor was discovered his prostate gland was removed and he was given intensive hormone treatment to control the metastasis. But his prognosis was not good, due to the time lapse.

All that glitters is not gold. All back pain with radiation to the leg is not indicative of a slipped disc. All back pain with spasms and apparent joint-grinding is not arthritis. Back pain can be helpful for singling out specific disorders. But it can also be misleading and therefore bad. Whichever, it should be enough to get you to a doctor as quickly as possible for a proper and correct diagnosis.

A rule of thumb that doctors use is, if a patient's back pain intensifies when lying down, suspect a tumor.

12.

Arthritis

Next to chronic back strain and to intervertebral disc degeneration, arthritis of the spine is probably the most frequent cause of chronic back pain. Yet it is not as frequent as people imagine. Indeed, it has been my experience that many more backache victims are walking around claiming they have arthritis than actually have it. Time after time patients come into my office complaining of arthritis in their backs. Someone told them they had it—a doctor, a chiropractor, a neighbor. They are then surprised to learn after my examination that they do not have arthritis at all, but some other disorder. Nevertheless people do suffer from arthritis of the back, so let's see what arthritis is and try to determine if this is the cause of your back pain.

Osteoarthritis

Osteoarthritis comprises by far the most common type of arthritis of the spine. It is a condition brought about mainly through wear-and-tear, and is usually hastened by prolonged faulty posture and chronic strain. It is not a disease in the sense that it is brought about by infection or by alteration of the basic metabolic processes It's simply a mechanical wearing-away of the joints of the spine.

Obviously the older we get, the more wear-and-tear occurs in our spine. Therefore osteoarthritis is more prevalent in older persons than younger.

Here is an example of how a typical case of osteoarthritis starts. It will usually begin with a person who is advancing in age, who has poor posture and who uses his back a great deal. As the discs in his spine gradually dry out (a normal part of the aging process), they become more easily subject

134

to trauma, and the normal uniform dispersion of pressure around the walls of the discs is diminished. Consequently, abnormal pressures are placed on certain portions of the discs.

I've described how discs protrude rearward into the spinal canal, causing the symptoms of slipped disc. But they can also protrude in other directions—either sideways or forward, or through the top or bottom plates of the disc capsule, which are connected to the vertebral bodies.

Let's say the bulge in this case is in the forward portion of the annulus fibrosus (see A of Fig. 14). Because the annulus in the forward portions of the discs is considerably thicker than in the rear, and because the *anterior longitudinal ligament* is stronger than the *posterior longitudinal ligament*, the discs will not rupture in this direction. They will, however, protrude against the *anterior longitudinal ligament*. When the pressure of a disc's bulge becomes great enough, it will lift this ligament off the front of the vertebral bodies, creating a gap between the forward edges of the vertebrae and the ligament to which they are normally attached. In this gap bone spurs grow from the vertebrae. These spurs

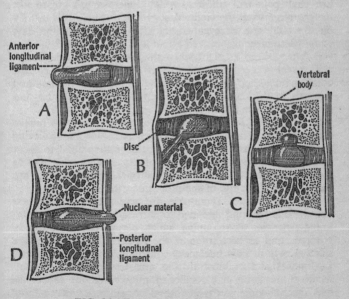

FIG. 14   Four types of disc protrusion.

may continue to grow towards each other. Eventually they will touch and then grow together, creating a spontaneous fusion of the vertebrae. Once this fusion has occurred no further motion will be able to take place at the joint.

Indeed, once the fusion has occurred the arthritic pain is likely to lessen. But while the bone spurs are growing and interfering with the natural configuration of the vertebral joints, pain is present.

This is the typical evolution of osteoarthritis, although it comes about in other ways too. No matter which way it comes, however, it is caused initially by the wear-and-tear process of the aging of the spine which invites such disorders. Osteoarthritis can involve the entire spine, but it most frequently occurs in those areas which have the most movement —the lumbar and cervical regions.

Unfortunately, medicine has yet to solve the problem of arthritis in general, and arthritis of the spine remains beyond cure. Yet it can be slowed down.

Diagnosis is reached on the basis of symptoms. X-ray findings and laboratory results. The principal symptoms are low back pain and stiffness, which generally are greatest in the morning when the victim first gets out of bed. It is usually on the mild side or even absent altogether during the day, once the sufferer has moved about a bit and warmed up, but will return again at night when the back is fatigued. X-rays will reveal a narrowing of the intervertebral joint spaces, bone spurs along the margins of the vertebral bodies, and sclerosis (a thickening and hardening) of the end plates that attach the discs to the vertebrae.

Treatment in the early stages is designed mainly to relieve the pain and spasms. This consists primarily of pain-relieving drugs and bed rest. If the symptoms do not respond to these measures, a surgical spinal fusion of the affected area may be the only corrective measure. But surgical spinal fusions are not performed for run-of-the-mill osteoarthritis.

Once the painful symptoms are under control, the best treatment is the kind designed to correct the obvious mechanical deficiencies of the spine which permit the condition to progress, and to take some of the stress off the spine in the affected region. This treatment consists of correcting postural weaknesses and building up the muscles around the region where the arthritis has developed so as to relieve the bones and discs of some of the abnormal pressures. By maintaining good posture while sitting, standing and sleeping, by avoiding unnecessary stresses on the back by bending and lifting, and, most importantly, by faithfully performing a daily program of back exercises, the pain and discomfort can be alleviated and the progress of the disease slowed.

Rheumatoid Arthritis

Rheumatoid arthritis is a disease, not a mechanical disorder, and is a good deal more serious than osteoarthritis. The disease can affect children as well as adults, and is progressive. It starts mainly in the large joints of the body but characteristically spreads to involve all joints, especially the hands, which become swollen, deformed and useless unless treatment is effective.

The disease usually involves the spine in its later stages. It differs from osteoarthritis in several ways, the most significant of which is that as it progresses, it causes *osteoporosis* (a thinning of the density of the bone) and fragility of the vertebrae.

The symptoms of such a disease are, obviously, severe pain and disability. If nothing else, it's fortunate that the condition is relatively rare, since nothing much can be done about it except to try to manage it through exercise and medication.

Another severe arthritic disease of the spine is one called *ankylosing spondylitis,* also known as Marie-Strumpel Disease. This disease produces bone between the intervertebral joints along the length of the spine until the spine becomes rigid. At the same time the dorsal or upper-back curve of the spine becomes exceedingly acute, causing the victim to be permanently bent.

This excessive bending of the spine can be alleviated somewhat by surgery. But since its treatment and therapy do not fall under the general scope of this book, I will not linger on it.

Gouty Arthritis

Here is another sure pain producer, although again, thankfully, it is not too frequent in the scheme of back disorders.

Gout is a metabolic disease, but it belongs here under the broad classification of arthritis. It is a disturbance of the metabolism involving uric acid, which is normally maintained at a specific level in the bloodstream. When it rises, usually because of some metabolic disturbance or imbalance in the system, uric acid crystals are formed. As these crystals flow through the blood they are deposited in and around the joints of the body. Classically they end up in the joints of the foot, particularly that of the big toe, creating a terribly painful condition.

Gout can also involve the spine, and when it does its symptoms usually mimic those of a slipped disc or other distressing disorders. X-rays of the spine will generally show nothing, but occasionally small flakes of what appear to be calcium can be seen in the intervertebral joints' peripheral tissues. They are not calcium particles but uric acid crystals. A definite diagnosis is easily made by conducting a uric acid blood test and a blood urea nitrogen test, which is an index of kidney function. If the uric acid level is high, the patient can be treated with the appropriate medication and his pain and other symptoms will subside.

Now that you are familiar with what arthritis of the spine really encompasses, I am sure that many of you have made up your minds that this is not what you have. I hope that those of you who have decided you don't have arthritis have also decided you would not like to develop it. Of course, you have no control over rheumatoid arthritis or Marie-Strumpel Disease. If you have developed gouty arthritis, which is basically a disease of males, it can be successfully treated with specific anti-gout medications. Osteoarthritis, on the other hand, which all of you will sooner or later get to one degree or another, can be controlled to a great extent through the pursuit of good posture and through the strengthening of your back muscles through exercise.

13.

General
Systemic Diseases

The Common Cold

If you're a steady watcher of television you've seen commercials for products which promise to "relieve the aches and pains of cold and flu." Whether the promises are fulfilled is not our concern here. What is our concern are the "aches and pains," especially those which arise in the back.

The common ordinary everyday cold or flu is a systemic disease—that is, it is an ailment that affects the entire system. Although a common cold is not a serious problem, it often does produce back pain and can lead to more serious back complications.

The kind of cold I'm talking about is brought about by a mild virus which gets into your bloodstream and creates conventional cold symptoms—sniffling, sore throat, and so on. Secondary symptoms which often occur are the familiar aches and pains all over your body—in your head, your shoulders, your back and your legs. These symptoms come about because your circulatory system spreads the virus throughout your body, lowering your overall resistance to the normal stresses and strains placed upon its muscles and joints. As your muscles are fatigued and weakened, mild spasm follows, and this explains why you get those aches and pains.

Now, an occasional cold or flu, although bothersome, is nothing to worry yourself about. But if you are the type of person who is subject to chronic colds, you might be in for back trouble unless you take certain precautions. The frequent incidence of colds will produce chronic fatigue of your

139

back muscles, weakening them and lessening their supportive capabilities. Such a situation is liable to get the "domino effect," which I mentioned earlier, into the act. It won't be long before the other structures in your back begin to weaken and the resulting complications develop. It is certainly no coincidence that some of the disc patients I have treated were people who suffered from chronic colds. Indeed, I have witnessed many instances when nothing more than a sneeze or cough has triggered a disc collapse.

It is of primary importance that cold sufferers strive extra hard to keep their back muscles strong and firm so as to counteract the effects of fatigue brought about by their colds.

And here's another point to keep in mind. Whenever you feel a sneeze or a cough coming on, *get your knees bent!* If you are standing, lean over and put your hands on your knees, much like a baseball fielder waiting for a ball to be hit to him. If you are in bed, raise your knees. When you sneeze or cough your entire body shakes and puts especially sudden and severe stresses on your lower back. These flexed positions immediately take some of the loads off your lower spine, where most sudden disc collapses occur.

The common cold is an example of a mild systemic disease which can create back problems. Other, much more serious systemic diseases such as rheumatoid arthritis, tumors and infections I have already discussed in previous chapters. These demand prolonged and intensive treatment and in some cases are beyond treatment. There is a third class of systemic diseases which produce back pain and which, though serious, are often responsive to treatment. These are metabolic and circulatory diseases, and it's time we took a brief look at them.

Metabolic Diseases

The processes of your metabolism—that is, the way your body functions—are all in delicate balance. One of the important components of your metabolism is your endocrine system, the system of glands which secrete hormones into your bloodstream. These various hormones control specific functions of the vital organs of your body.

The endocrine system is mysterious and fascinating and makes one marvel once again at the complexity of the bodies with which we are endowed. But like everything else, no matter how good the system is, things do go wrong, and when the endocrine balance is upset trouble follows.

Take, for instance, the master gland—the pituitary—which controls the function of all the other glands in the endocrine system. One of the things it produces by itself is a growth hormone. Too little of this hormone results in a dwarf, too much in a giant. Both are abnormal and both are likely to have back problems, particularly the giant, whose vertebrae are large and somewhat flattened. Whereas the pituitary dwarf is generally well proportioned skeletally, the pituitary giant is not—he has huge hands and feet, a tremendous jaw, and large, almost elephantine ears. All this just from too much of one hormone from a tiny gland.

Another imbalance occurs when there is a lack of insulin produced by the pancreas. The result is diabetes, a serious but treatable metabolic disease. And so the list goes on.

There are three endocrinological disturbances that affect the bones of the spine and are devilishly capable of producing back pain. These are *hyperthyroidism, hyperparathyroidism,* and *hyperadrenalism,* also known as *Cushing's Syndrome.*

The thyroid is a gland in the neck which controls the rate of your metabolic functions. When your thyroid becomes hyperactive you tend to become very nervous and to burn off a lot of energy. When your thyroid is underactive you tend to become sluggish, to have less energy. Your skin becomes dry and you are likely to gain weight unaccountably.

One of the additional adverse effects of hyperthyroidism is that sometimes the metabolism is speeded up to such an extent that calcium is pulled out of the bones, especially those of the spine. When this happens the vertebrae lose some of their density, as in osteoporosis (about which more in the next chapter), and they become fragile and liable to collapse.

The parathyroid glands are four small glands located, two apiece, on either side of the thyroid. They have a specific effect on the metabolism of calcium. When these glands become overactive calcium is, again, pulled out of the bones, but not in a uniform fashion. Irregular gaps are created in the bone and these spaces fill up with fibrous tissue. These spaces resemble tumors on X-ray, and before this condition was understood many patients would have tumors diagnosed only to discover after surgery that a hyperactive parathyroid was their problem.

Hyperadrenalism, or Cushing's Syndrome, occurs when there is too much cortisone in the system. Cortisone is produced by the adrenal glands, which lie near each kidney. If the outer portion of one or more of these glands becomes too active, that is, if it secretes more cortisone than the system can handle, osteoporosis will result, with all its symptoms and dangers for the spine.

There are other metabolic diseases which exist besides endocrinological disturbances. One worth touching on here has to do with a breakdown in a chemical process of the body. It's called *ochronosis*, and it occurs when a substance known as *homogentisic acid* is not metabolized properly and is allowed to circulate in the bloodstream. Its presence in the blood, like excess uric acid, is abnormal. It has a tendency to become lodged in the body's cartilage tissue (because it turns black when exposed to air, a person with this problem may develop black ears). Its significance for this book is that it also is deposited in the intervertebral discs of the spine, part of which are cartilage, and produces degeneration and pain.

A much more significant and frequent disease of the spinal bones is *Paget's Disease*, named, as you've probably guessed by now, after the doctor who first described it. It is also known as *osteitis deformans*. It is not an infection, it is not a tumor, it is not really even a true metabolic disease. It can involve all the bones of the body, but often occurs in the bones of the spine.

What happens when it occurs in the spine is that one or more vertebral bones begin to proliferate—that is, they enlarge in all directions. As the vertebrae thicken (the disease is usually limited to the vertebrae of the lower spine and to the pelvic bones), the little holes, or *foramina*, through which the nerve roots pass to and from the spinal cord, narrow. When there is sufficient narrowing or reduction in the size of the foramina, the nerve roots are likely to be compressed and irritated, which causes localized deep-seated low-back pain as well as pain in the buttocks and down the backs of the thighs. The pain is more or less constant, but from time to time can become more intense, whether in bed or out.

Since the cause of Paget's Disease is unknown, there is no clinical remedy for it, but diagnosis is fairly easy. The disease shows up readily on X-rays, and is confirmed by certain blood tests, especially the *enzyme alkaline phosphatase* test. Surgery is the only way we have at present of relieving the compression of the nerve roots caused by the disease. This consists of the procedure known as *laminectomy*, which means removing the rear portion—the posterior neural arch—of the affected vertebra to relieve the pressure on the nerve roots.

Circulatory Diseases

The simple facts of blood circulation are that the arteries in our bodies take fresh oxygenated blood from our hearts to all our body cells and tissues. Without oxygen none of these cells and tissues can survive. Our brain cells are most susceptible to decreased oxygen supply and will die after only four minutes of oxygen deprivation. Muscles, bones and peripheral nerve tissues and cells, on the other hand, can last an hour or more without oxygen.

Once fresh blood is delivered by our arteries and employed by our cells and tissues, it becomes, so to speak, used blood. The veins in our bodies pick up the used blood, which now has a high carbon dioxide content, and return the blood to our hearts, which then recycle it through our lungs to rid it of its carbon dioxide wastes and infuse it with fresh oxygen (if such is available in these days of increasing air pollution).

That, in a nutshell, is our circulatory system. But like everything else, it can go wrong and cause a variety of problems throughout our bodies. Our backs are not immune from such problems.

Two things can go wrong with our circulatory system: either the arteries are for some reason unable to deliver fresh blood in the required amounts to its natural destinations, or else the veins are for some reason unable to return the used blood to the factory—the heart—for recycling.

Let us assume for our purposes here that in either case the heart is not the culprit in the breakdown of the system, although it sometimes is. If the heart is working normally as an efficient pump, clean fresh blood pours through the arteries. But if there is an obstruction in one or more of the arteries—a clot (*embolus*)—the blood will not be able to get through. Or if the clot is partial, only an insufficient flow of blood is possible. Thus a partial or complete arterial embolism is one possible cause of a breakdown in the circulatory system.

Another is a result of the arterial pipe being narrowed, as happens in *arteriosclerosis*, or hardening of the arteries. Again, the proper flow of blood is diminished, and the vital parts of the body supplied by the affected artery are deprived of their needed blood feed.

When the cells of muscle and other body tissue are suddenly and completely deprived of blood, they will die after an hour or two. If the supply of blood is diminished, but is still sufficient to keep the cells alive, the tissues will continue to live but will have no tolerance for activity. Activity, therefore, even the normal activity of supporting a particular body structure, will produce pain.

I have a friend whose father complained of increasing leg and back pain over a period of two years. He was a very active man who, after two years of seeing different doctors, was confined to bed, the diagnosis being that he had two or three slipped discs. A more accurate diagnosis finally determined that his problem was not in his discs—although the pain symptoms mimicked disc pain—but in his leg arteries. Indeed, he had several blood clots in these arteries which created insufficient blood supply to his thigh and calf muscles and produced leg and lower back pains similar to disc pain. Surgery was performed, the clots were removed, and a few months later the patient was leading a perfectly normal life.

Breakdowns in the veins are generally less serious than arterial obstructions, but can also produce severe pain. Varicose veins are often the source of leg pain that can radiate into the back and cause mistaken diagnoses. *Thrombophlebitis,* or inflammations of the veins, is another villain. When the veins become inflamed a slow-down in the return of used blood to the heart is created. As the blood flow backs up it begins to stagnate. Clots form, which then may break off and be carried to the heart and lungs, causing damage there.

This is another example of why it is so important for a doctor to be complete in his approach to a diagnosis of back pain. If circulatory insufficiency in the legs and lower back produce back pain, and if doctors fail to take into account the possibility of circulatory problems as a possible source of such pain, mistaken diagnoses and incorrect treatment will be the result.

14.

The Aging Process and Hormonal Changes

The process of aging has come under especially close scrutiny by the scientific world during the last decade or so. Huge sums of money have been spent by government and private interests to support research into this area.

The two great questions about the aging process which science is trying to answer are: "Why do we grow old?" and "How do we grow old?" In response to the first query we can only restate the obvious—that no form of life is permanent. And with respect to the second, we do not even have an obscure answer.

Yet we do know that one of the primary characteristics of aging is that the body's tissues tend to lose their water content and dry out. This loss of fluid substance is of particular significance when it comes to the back. Indeed, the spine starts to age earlier than other parts of the body. Your intervertebral discs, for instance, begin to lose their water content when you are still in your twenties. Aside from the possible disc problems that arise as a result of injury, general back instability and disease, the discs are subject to the degenerative effects of aging.

It is important to remember that the discs constitute approximately 25 percent of the entire length of the spinal column. As the discs lose their water content they shrink. As the years go by they grow even smaller, compressing and gradually losing their shock-absorbing capability. Motion between the vertebral bodies becomes diminished and greater stresses and loads are placed on their supporting ligaments. A chronic straining condition begins. The strains are in turn transferred to the vertebrae themselves as ligamentous tissue is pulled away from the bones. The bones react by producing bone spurs to fill the gaps left by the stretched ligaments. All of this because the discs lose their water content.

So disc degeneration associated with the aging process leads to a loss of height in the spinal column and consequently loss of overall height. This leads to greater stresses on the ligaments connecting the discs and the vertebrae. And this leads to what we have already described as osteoarthritis.

You can see, then, that hardly anyone will escape osteoarthritis. However, this is a condition which, although practically inevitable in all of us, need not be painful or debilitating provided that the spine's supporting structures are kept in good condition from an early age. It is the combination of poor posture, weak back muscles, and the natural and normal degeneration of the discs that makes for painful osteoarthritis in our later years. As in everything else having to do with the back, the back is only as good as its weakest link. And the more weak links there are, the sooner will the back prove painful and troublesome.

Osteoporosis

I've already mentioned osteoporosis in the last chapter when I described one of the serious effects of Cushing's Syndrome, or hyperadrenalism. Cushing's Syndrome is rare, but aging is not—we all grow old. One of the unfortunate things about growing old is that with it often comes osteoporosis.

If you had any course in Latin during your school days you might guess that the word "osteoporosis" means a "porousness of the bone." This pretty well describes what happens when osteoporosis occurs: the bones become porous, which means they lose their density. Many doctors prefer the word "osteopoenia" because it more aptly describes the problem, which is a decrease in the substance of the bone.

Whichever word is used, you can be sure the problem it relates to is not a pleasant one. Nor is the back pain it produces.

In order to better understand the concept of osteoporosis you must realize that the bone in your body is not inert or inactive—a common misconception that many people hold. Your bones are as alive as the rest of you. They play two important metabolic roles in the function of your system—they produce blood cells and they store minerals, especially calcium. Portions of your bones are constantly dissolving and new bone is being produced to replace it. It has been calculated that every bone in an active person's body is completely replaced over a seven year period. This is quite an achievement. Indeed, no other tissue in your body has such excellent regenerative powers except for your skin. And when bones fracture, they heal back together again without leaving scars. Not even skin can do that.

Consider, then, the bones of your body as another vital organ system like that of your liver, spleen or heart. Your bones actively participate in your body's metabolism.

Bone is composed of two components. One is the matrix, which is a protein substance that acts as a kind of template upon which calcium salts are deposited to form the bone. The other is an intercellular substance which fills the miscroscopic spaces within the hardened calcium and acts as a sort of cement to hold the entire affair together. The protein matrix on which the bone forms through the action of the calcium salts is produced by bone cells called "osteoblasts." Other cells, called "osteoclasts," are responsible for resorbing or removing bone that is dead or non-functioning. A balance exists between these two cell factors, one producing bone while the other reduces it. The appearance and strength of bone is undisturbed during this continual process. But when the osteoclasts resorb more bone than the osteoblasts are able to produce, there will be a decrease in bone substance and osteoporosis results.

Why this happens we do not know, but happen it does. And where it is most likely to happen is in the bones of the spine, the vertebral bodies. Although we don't know for sure, we can make a good guess as to why osteoporosis affects the bones of the back sooner than any other in the body.

Bone is not only made up of two basic component substances, it also has two characteristics. We might call these characteristics hard and soft. The deep interior of any bone is relatively soft when compared to the exterior, which is hard. This soft interior is known as the "cancellous" portion of the bone, while the hard exterior is known as the "cortical" portion. The cancellous portion of bone, being softer, is also more "alive" in the sense of storing minerals and producing blood. In other words it takes a greater role in the body's metabolic function than does the harder exterior portion. Because of this the cancellous portion of bone is more subject to metabolic imbalances, especially those having to do with the endocrine system and its production of hormones.

Now, the bones of the spine, the vertebrae, are much more cancellous than they are cortical—that is, they are formed mostly of the softer bone tissue and have very little hard bone in their make-up. Therefore, they are that much more likely to be affected by changes in the metabolism than other bones of the body. And again, although we do not know for sure, all evidence seems to point to the fact that osteoporosis is caused by specific hormonal imbalances, both those associated with disease and those associated with aging.

Although osteoporosis occurs with certain metabolic diseases, as described in the previous chapter, it also occurs naturally with specific hormonal changes that come about as a result of aging and as a result, in women, of the menopause.

By far the most frequent incidence of osteoporosis occurs in older women who have gone through the menopause. If you are a woman in your late forties or early fifties and start having bad backache, you can start thinking about osteoporosis. If the pain seems to go deep and is continual, you and your doctor can think about osteoporosis even more. By this time the situation calls for an X-ray examination, especially if you can't remember any good reason behind your pain, such as a fall or a heavy strain, that might otherwise explain it.

If you have osteoporosis the X-ray film will reveal the true state of affairs. Almost any technician with even limited experience can identify the characteristically indistinct, hazy appearance of the vertebrae which is indicative of osteoporosis.

What it all means is that your vertebrae have begun to lose their normal density and are growing weaker. If allowed to progress the condition can lead to compressed, collapsed or crushed vertebrae.

The evident fact is that as a result of your having passed through the menopause the production of certain of your female sexual hormones has been decreased. This is logical—your reproductive system, having no longer any need of the necessary hormones required to keep it active, signals your ovaries to stop producing the necessary hormones. This most likely triggers an hormonal imbalance in your body which in turn brings about osteoporosis.

The treatment, despite the uncertainty as to the exact cause of the disease, is more or less standard. And unfortunately, it is more or less standardly unsuccessful. The generally accepted procedure calls for periodic doses of the male and female hormones—testosterone and estrogen—along with calcium and vitamin D. All, usually, to no avail.

Although progressive, the back pain associated with postmenopausal osteoporosis can be slowed down through exercise and the strengthening of the spine's supportive muscles. The same goes for ordinary senile osteoporosis—the condition associated with old age.

In senile osteoporosis a different group of hormones are used in treatment, along with calcium and vitamin D. And the results are usually the same as with the postmenopausal condition—which is to say no positive results at all. The simple unhappy fact is that up to the present time neither surgical nor clinical treatments of this disease have been very effective. When and if one or more vertebral bodies collapse as a result of excessive thinning of the bone, light back supports in the form of braces may be necessary. Bed rest is not very effective because once the vertebral bodies begin to deteriorate, disuse accelerates the process. Bed rest in the elderly, especially, must be kept at a minimum due to its adverse effects on their minds and bodies. Indeed, bed rest has no place in the treatment of osteoporosis because it tends to further weaken the back's supporting muscles.

The only effective therapy is through exercise designed to improve muscle tone and strength and to maintain as much compensatory motion in the hip joints as possible. The purpose of both is to relieve the stresses on the weakened vertebral bodies and joints.

A by-product of osteoporosis is a condition known as "ballooned discs." Osteoporosis will sufficiently weaken the vertebral bodies to allow the pressure of the intervertebral discs to expand the discs through the upper and lower plates, by which they are connected to the bodies, and into the bodies themselves. This will only happen when the disc still has its elastic gelatinous nucleus. If the disc's nucleus has lost its integrity or dried out sufficiently, this is not likely to occur. Rather the opposite will happen—disc collapse.

To summarize this chapter, osteoarthritis and osteoporosis are both pain-producing disorders of the back which are part of the aging process. In addition, osteoporosis is probably due to endocrinological changes that occur in the body due to hormonal changes resulting either from metabolic disease or from the aging process itself. These conditions lead to loss of overall height, to increased curvature of the spine through disc or vertebrae degeneration, and in severe cases to the collapse of vertebrae themselves. To date we are helpless to prevent the occurrence of these disorders and are ill equipped to cure them. However, we are able to modify them by means of exercise designed to relieve the normal loads and stresses placed on the affected spinal parts, and are therefore capable of relieving the pain and disability they produce.

15.

Pregnancy

It never fails to depress me when I watch a pregnant woman, who should be filled with the joy and excitement of having a new life forming in her womb, let those wonderful feelings become compromised by the presence of nagging backache.

I do not have actual statistics on the number of pregnant women in this country who have chronic back pain, but my medical experience tells me they are innumerable. The saddest part of this is that the back pain of pregnancy is avoidable in the great majority of cases. Furthermore, when the back pain of pregnancy is ignored it can and often does lead to chronic life-long back problems. My files are filled with cases of female patients who have told me that the onset of their back symptoms coincided with their first pregnancies.

What makes pregnant women so susceptible to back pain? The answer would seem to be obvious. Indeed, it seems so obvious that most pregnant women I see tend to accept their back pain as an inevitable consequence of their becoming pregnant, just as they accept morning sickness and breast enlargement. I know many women who, in the advanced stages of their pregnancy, are likely to say, "Well, look at me—how can I expect not to have a backache with this big stomach of mine?" What they are doing when they say this is rationalizing their back pain, using their pregnancy as an excuse to grin and bear it.

But must they bear it? I don't think so, and the success I've had in reversing back pain in pregnant women bears me out. Again, like everything else having to do with strain-induced back pain, a simple understanding of how it comes about can go a long way toward alleviating it.

Three Structural Factors

As I've said, the reason for back pain in pregnancy would *seem* to be pretty obvious and inevitable. But let's take a closer look and see if that's true. If you are pregnant and have back pain, and assuming you do not have an organic disorder in your back, the likelihood is that you're a victim of three structural factors which join together to produce your pain.

The first arises in the early stages of your pregnancy. Before your abdomen begins to protrude and before you start to gain weight, you will feel tired, require a great deal of sleep, and tend to become less active. These normal symptoms of pregnancy are associated with the hormonal changes that take place within your body. If you've already got poor posture (which also seems to be the norm these days), that, coupled with the increasing weakening and fatigue of your back muscles, will produce minor nagging backache in the lower region of your spine.

Later, as the fetus grows, your abdomen's protuberance increases and you gain weight. Your posture and back muscles become more relaxed, and the forces of gravity increase the lumbar curve of your spine, creating a swayback condition. As weight and frontal protuberance increase in front of your lumbar spine, the stresses on your lower back are further intensified. Your weakened back muscles fatigue more easily, and rather than take up the full loads, they protest. The protest comes in the form of increased pain as a result of spasm.

Towards the end of your pregnancy something new happens. Special hormones are secreted within your body which are designed to loosen the ligaments which hold your pelvis together. The ligaments become lax in preparation for the distension of your pelvis, which occurs as you approach your delivery. This relaxing of the ligaments is not selective; therefore, all the supporting structures of your lower spine are involved. As the ligaments relax their normal tensions your lower spine loses some of its support and becomes even more pronounced in its abnormal curve, further straining your back muscles and increasing your back pain.

I'm sure you all are familiar with the classic picture of the very pregnant woman pushing a stroller down the street. One hand is on the stroller's handle, the other buried in the small of her back. The expression on her face says, "Oh, my aching back!" I know an awful lot of women who identify with that picture—needlessly, I might add.

Most pregnant women complain of backache, but there are many who complain of pain in their legs as well. The majority of such leg pain is due to plain muscle fatigue or to congestion of the veins. But a certain percentage of it is due to pressure on the lumbar nerve roots, especially the two lowest ones in the lumbar spine which pass through the psoas muscle. If the baby is large and lies on these nerves, they become compressed and irritated, causing pain to shoot down the legs. After delivery this pain subsides without recurrence. But in other cases, if the radiating pain is due to a herniated disc which has collapsed as a result of the added stresses placed upon it, it does not subside after birth. It lingers on to plague the mother. This, then, becomes a chronic problem.

Indeed, many different organic back problems that arise in women later in their lives can be traced to the structural weaknesses that developed in their backs as a result of pregnancy. The saddest thing about this is that the entire syndrome—both the back pain of pregnancy and the later complications—could have been so easily avoided with a few minutes a day of exercise during pregnancy.

Pregnancy obviously adds great stress to the lower spine. In order to counteract these forces a pregnant woman must concentrate on establishing good posture and on doing a program of exercises to strengthen the supporting muscles of her back. Most obstetricians advise their patients very well in this regard and many hospitals have exercise programs for pregnant women which are often open to the expectant fathers as well.

However, once-a-week exercising is not enough. Good advice is not enough. The responsibility eventually rests with the woman herself. Like so many other things in life, you have to work for your rewards. A woman who expects to sail through her pregnancy without working to counteract the ill effects on her back is merely conducting an exercise in self-delusion. The penalties she will suffer are great. Conversely, the rewards of diligent attention to her back are equally great.

The exercises a pregnant woman can do are no different than those which will help anyone else with a weak back. They are simple, easy, and healthful. They should be pursued

diligently and should become as much a part of her day as
her hygiene habits. Once embarked upon, the decrease and
eventual absence of severe back pain will be sufficient motivation to convince her to stick to them, even in the face of
boredom.

The Coccyx—A Special Problem

That little vestigial tail of ours at the bottom of our spine,
which we usually never notice unless we fall directly on it,
can also create painful symptoms during pregnancy, especially during the delivery and immediately thereafter.

The ligaments which are attached to your coccyx help support your pelvis. Great stress is applied to this area during
labor and actual delivery, and many women become aware of
excruciating pain at the base of the spine after they've been
wheeled from the delivery room. They are unable to lie comfortably on their backs and will constantly strain to take the
pressure off the area.

The treatment consists simply of avoiding pressure on the
painful spot, and this is usually done through the use of an
inflated rubber "donut." Warm soaks also help, but baths are
usually not permitted until six weeks after delivery. An injection of Cortisone and Xylocaine directly into the painful
site results in more immediate relief and is perfectly safe.
After awhile the pain subsides and rarely, if ever, occurs unless there is a subsequent injury to the coccyx.

Rare Disorders

Practically all pregnancy-associated back pain comes about
as a result of the factors which I have just related, and the
back pain is relievable through improvement of posture and
strengthening of the back muscles.

Nevertheless, there are two organic disorders associated
with pregnancy which, though rare, are worth a paragraph
or two. This is not to say they are caused by pregnancy. Indeed, we do not know what causes them. One is seen almost
exclusively in pregnant women, while the second can occur
in other situations as well.

The first is *osteomalacia*. A first cousin of osteoporosis, it
means a softening of the bone. Actually this disease, which

attacks pretty nearly any bone in the pelvis as well as the lower lumbar vertebrae, is a form of adult rickets. It stems from the same kind of vitamin deficiency responsible for rickets in children. The pain of osteomalacia is similar to that of osteoporosis.

A diagnosis of osteomalacia in pregnant women might compel a Caesarian delivery, because the weak, softened bones of the pelvic outlet, through which the baby must pass, may have been deformed, twisted, shifted or bent so as to make normal birth passage impossible.

Just as an increasing understanding of the nutritional factors involved has almost entirely eliminated rickets as a disease of children, so proper diet, containing the necessary components, such as Vitamin D and calcium, has practically eliminated osteomalacia in pregnant women. This is one of the reasons your obstetrician stresses proper diet so often. And since it is a diet-deficiency disease, osteomalacia is now rare among American women, who are generally well fed.

The other organic disorder associated with pregnancy is *osteitis condensans*. Unlike osteomalacia, there is no known cure for this disease but, again, it is relatively rare. It seems to be closely associated with pregnancy in the sense that pregnancy seems to aggravate the condition, and a well-developed case can produce considerably more pain than either osteoporosis or osteomalacia.

As osteitis condensans progresses, the affected bones— usually the two ilia (which form the sides of the pelvis)— gradually grow harder and harder as more and more calcium salts are accumulated. The bones become stonelike, lacking the normal cellular composition of healthy bone, and the condition seems to worsen with each successive pregnancy.

In severe attacks the doctor can only offer painkillers of some kind and advise avoidance of further childbearing. I emphasize again that this disease is rare and, as far as we know, is not caused by pregnancy. In fact its cause is a mystery, and we can only guess that it resides somewhere in the metabolism.

Just as it is a wise father who knows his children, it is a wise mother who, early in her pregnancy, understands the relationship between pregnancy and back pain.

16.

Referred
Pain

Up until now I have been talking about the pain you get when
something goes wrong with your back. This ought to tell
the whole story, but it doesn't. There is a lot of back pain
you can get when there's absolutely nothing at all wrong with
your back except for some neurological short circuits.

These backaches, your doctor will tell you, are due to referred causes. That means the cause of your pain is elsewhere
than in your back. But because of the common pathways
your back nerves share with nerves supplying other parts of
your body, the pain is interpreted by your brain as arising in
your back.

You have already seen how enormously intricate your
nervous system is. Through this complex network every organ, bone, limb, joint, muscle and gland in your body, right
down to the last bit of cell tissue, is responsively linked together. Except for twelve sets of principal nerves running
from your brain, all the rest, from the tip of your toes to the
top of your head, ultimately tie in with your spine.

A large part of the business of keeping you alive is carried
over these nerve circuits in a completely automatic way,
without deliberate thinking on your part. I've already mentioned that you cannot will your heart to slow down or your
kidney to stop functioning. It's impossible to imagine just what
kind of constant, detailed brainwork it would take to keep
such things as your digestion, lungs, kidneys and liver on the
job if these automatic nerve functions didn't tend to them.

Nevertheless, while they are primarily automatic, it is also
true that your conscious thinking can and does affect the

working of these nerves. You can not escape reaction to the endless stream of impressions, thoughts, memories, emotions and other outside stimuli that come to you through your senses. The reactions you experience from these will inevitably have an effect on your autonomic nervous system.

For example, you may choose to direct your thinking where you shouldn't. The resulting blush that brightens your cheeks will betray your indiscretion. Or the sight of an accident victim, blood all over him, can spoil your appetite or bring an involuntary gasp to your lips. The horror and fear produced by the sight may even induce nausea and vomiting, or provoke you to faint into unconsciousness.

So you see, then, although the autonomic nervous system acts according to the strict rules built into it, it can be affected by outside stimuli. It can likewise be affected by a certain amount of neurological confusion which is built into our system due to the incredibly complex network of nerve pathways and to the "mixing" of nerves.

For the most part, day in and day out, second by second, your nervous system keeps you functioning with a minimum of fuss. The proper control centers located in your brain and spinal cord get immediate and complete information about each of your organs and body parts. At the same time the necessary orders for the continuation of proper functioning shoot back from the control centers to the various organs and parts.

But there are times when the signals get mixed up and a disorder in one part of the body will cause pain symptoms in another. A classic example of this is heart attack—a heart attack will often produce pain down the left arm. Gall bladder afflictions often manifest themselves by producing pain in the right shoulder. A classic orthopaedic example of pain referral is when a young child is brought into my office complaining of intense pain in the knee; examination and X-ray reveal that he really has a hip problem, but because his knee shares a common nerve with his hip, the pain appears to settle there.

There are several examples of organic disorders in other parts of the body which cause pain in the back. Stomach ulcers and other ailments of the digestive system will often cause back pain. So will kidney infections. In women lower back pain can be caused by tipped uterus or infections of the ovaries or fallopian tubes. Many women commonly get backache with the onset of their menstrual periods, as well. In men prostate gland infections frequently manifest themselves in low back pain. And of course tumors and abscesses in the general area of the bowels and intestines can cause back pain in both sexes, not to mention the circulatory problems of the legs which I've already discussed.

The presence of all these causes of back pain which do not reside in the back can be detected by the usual careful medical history, meticulous physical examination, and confirmatory laboratory tests. By remembering to think about these possible causes of back pain, a doctor can then eliminate them on the road to a true diagnosis, unless, of course, one or more of the tests returns positive findings.

Referred pain works the other way, too. That is, a pain in the leg may have its cause in the back. This type of pain, which we call sciatica, has already been discussed, so we won't linger on it here.

I can give you a very personal example of how referred pain works. I mentioned at the beginning of this book that I had suffered for many years with chronic severe back pain but had conquered it through back-strengthening exercises which I diligently pursued. Not too long ago, after a particularly strenuous day in the operating room and in my office, I experienced some rather sharp pain in my right mid-back region. I was sure I had pulled a muscle or strained myself in some way during my day's activities, but I had an even deeper fear that perhaps my old pain was about to reappear.

My initial reaction was to try to dissipate the pain by moving my arm around. That didn't work. So I exercised my upper back for a few days. This had always been helpful to me in the past when I suffered specific muscle strains, but the pain still did not go away. So then I decided to give my back a few days of rest in the hopes that the pain would subside spontaneously. Still no luck.

During the following weekend, in fact, my back pain increased in intensity and I began to have a low fever. Finally I did the wisest thing—what I should have done in the first place. I stopped treating myself and visited an internist. He examined me, took X-rays, and discovered that I had a case of viral pneumonia. This is a mild form of pneumonia, what old-time doctors used to call "walking pneumonia." It causes very little coughing and only a low-grade fever, but it does produce localized back pain similar to that of a strained muscle.

Well, I was sent home and stayed in bed for a few days. My pneumonia got better and my back pain subsided. Actually I could have shortened the whole process, which by now had spread over two weeks, by consulting the internist sooner. But, well—

There are two morals to this anecdote. One is that pneumonia can cause referred pain to the back, and that is one of the points of this chapter. The other moral is that the doctor who treats himself has a fool for a patient!

17.

Emotional and Psychological Factors

By now you've learned what a marvelously complex mechanism your back is. It is an amazingly durable hunk of machinery, ready to serve the purposes of a furniture mover or a banker, a ditch digger or a stenographer equally well. Yet it is also a highly sensitive mechanism. And unless you're looking for trouble, you'll give your back a chance to adjust to the different roles it is designed to play in your life.

Along with the physical work it does, your back unmistakably reflects your state of mind at any given moment. The inner tensions and turmoils caused by various stresses to which everyone is susceptible—whether they be major, such as a serious illness to a loved one, or minor, such as "should we paint the room red or blue?"—can effect our entire physical well being and especially our muscles.

Thus, when you are tense and anxious, your muscles become tight; and because your back muscles are subject to constant fatigue, they are particularly vulnerable to these inner tensions. Very much like an expressive face, our muscles, particularly our back muscles, reflect the state of our inner beings.

Emotional stress or tension is as tiring as physical stress or tension. Your entire body can be affected by emotional fatigue, which causes your muscles to grow tense and contract. Since your back muscles are constantly working while you are sitting or standing, they are likely to bear the brunt of your emotional fatigue sooner than others.

Fatigue, Stress and Tension

I believe that we all have various "stress organs." We all react to stress in different ways, and each of us tends to have one organ that reacts more strongly than others. Some of us develop heart problems as a result of stress, others stomach ulcers, others spastic colons, others migraine headaches, others backaches. There always seems to be one organ in our body which reacts to prolonged tension quicker than any others. For unknown reasons which are probably related to heredity, these organs bear most of the brunt of prolonged stress and tension.

When we say people are "uptight," we mean that literally. Gastric juices increase. Blood vessels go into spasm, particularly the coronary vessels of the heart. Muscles clench and contract, especially the back muscles. When tension is allowed to persist unabated, the stress continues to build up and finally something has to give.

Many of you have possibly heard the term "ulcer personality." This is a phrase internists and other doctors use to describe people with certain characteristics who, because they have these characteristics, are likely to develop ulcers, or, having developed them, are likely to re-develop them once they're cured—unless they are able to remove these characteristics from their personalities. An "ulcer personality" is usually one who keeps everything in, who worries but shares his worries with no one else, and who finds it difficult to both laugh and cry.

There is also such a thing as a backache personality, and the characteristics are similar, though more diverse and more widespread. The way a person copes with the stresses and tensions of modern life definitely plays an important role in his susceptibility to back pain. This includes just about anyone who is trying to get somewhere in this world. Take Harold Dennis, for instance.

Harry was blessed with a combination of brain and brawn. As a child growing up in rural Pennsylvania, he demonstrated great abilities on the athletic fields and in the classroom. He was always first, first in his class and captain of the football, baseball, and basketball teams in his senior year in high school. He thrived on the accolades of his friends and teachers, and worked even harder to reach greater heights. He won a scholarship to a large prestigious college where football was a major sport. For the first time, Harry was up against players that had more skill and ability than he did. However, his intense desire and his ability to drive himself to the limit propelled him forward so that he achieved great prominence as a player. He did not neglect his studies either, and he graduated with honors.

After graduation he attended law school and then finally joined a prestigious law firm in New York City. By this time Harry had married and had had two small children. He lived in the suburbs and commuted daily to his office. As usual for him, he worked long hard hours but was very productive. He was given greater responsibility and more difficult cases, all of which required more and more time. He had less time for his family and less time for himself. He stopped exercising, ate too much, and became overweight. At thirty-eight he was a big, somewhat paunchy man who still looked very fit and able, but who already had telltale bags under his eyes and the look of gray fatigue on his face from lack of fresh air and adequate rest. But he kept pushing. His family complained that they hardly saw him. He spent hours flying around the country; often he would fly back and forth to Europe twice in one week. He tried to ignore the fatigue, he told himself it was part of the job, but he was aware of tension in the muscles of his neck and lower back. Walking up three flights of stairs left him breathless. He kept telling himself that he would begin exercising again, get back into shape; but somehow he never got started. Then one day, after a heavy summer rain storm, he tried to open a tight window. It resisted his first efforts so he bent over and "put his back into it." Suddenly he experienced the most excruciating shock of pain across his lower back. He could hardly breathe, let alone straighten up. His wife had to help him to bed and to lie down. The acute spasm subsided, but as soon as he tried to move the pain would recur. After two days, he finally came to my office, when the pain still persisted.

I examined him carefully and gently because sudden movements were still painful. X-rays of his lower back were normal. He had no evidence of sciatic symptoms or herniated disc. I explained this to him. He was confused and upset. "Are you telling me that I have nothing wrong with my back?" "No, Harry," I replied. "What I am telling you is that your back and stomach muscles are weak, that your hamstrings are tight, that you are fat and overweight, and that you are way out of shape!"

"But Doctor," he protested, "I did not do anything strenuously. I simply bent and lifted up a tight window. My God, I used to lift two hundred pounds without any effort."

"Yes, Harry," I acknowledged, "that is true, but that was many years ago. You have let yourself go. You have stopped exercising, you have become soft and flabby, and although your mind may be willing, your body is not able." Explaining the problem to Harry took as much time as the examination itself. Convincing him that an exercise program (as outlined in Chapter 19 in this book) would help was even more difficult. Attempting to change his life-style was impossible. However, he was intelligent, he had had a good scare, and so he was willing to work at the exercises and slightly modify his work and eating habits. Over the next few days, the spasm in his back subsided. He began the exercise program, once in the morning when he awoke and again at night when he went to sleep. As he progressed, he discovered that the exercises not only strengthened his back, but that they relieved the tension in his muscles. His flexibility returned. He was able to sit in a chair or drive in a car without being stiff and achy. He resumed squash, playing three times a week regularly. He ate normally but sensibly. His waistline thinned. His tailor enjoyed taking in his clothes. Harry discovered that he could work hard, achieve a great deal, and still be healthy and well.

But Harry was only human, and after a year of feeling very well, he began to miss an occasional morning of exercises. The work days became longer, the squash infrequent. Soon the back exercise program ceased entirely and his weight increased. One early morning, I received an urgent phone call.

"Doctor, it's Harry Dennis. I am in severe pain, my back is killing me, and I can't move."

"Harry," I asked, "when did you stop your exercise program?"

There was a moment or two of silence and then, "How did you know?" he asked. "Yes, I stopped four months ago."

That was typical. So often, you work to strengthen your muscles and then allow them to weaken by resuming poor patterns of behavior, and once again you find yourself in trouble and pain.

Well, Harry learned his lesson the second time. He has continued faithfully with his back exercise program and I have not had any further urgent calls.

Harry Dennis is just one of thousands of typical "backache personalities" I could parade before you. If he had let his condition develop into a chronic one the likelihood is that he would have eventually developed a serious disorder of the spine. Fortunately for him his competitiveness, as with everything else in his life, drove him to overcome his condition so that it would not become chronic. How about you?

I have a cat at home which almost daily demonstrates this early trait of man. Every time a strange dog comes into the house the cat will either face up to the dog or flee under a bed, depending on the size of the dog. In either case the cat will react with a physical action. If the dog chases her and traps her in a corner, she'll go through the familiar cat reactions—arching her back, swelling her tail, spitting and snarling, and so on. But this fierce tension, and the psychological stresses it places on the cat, last only for a few minutes at most. Sooner or later the cat, in her fury, will either force the dog to retreat, allowing her to find another hiding place, or else will attack the dog in a blur of claws and snarls until the dog decides it would be better off elsewhere. Once the threat is removed from the house, the cat will be back in my lap purring contentedly.

Dr. Hans Selye, in 1946, described the way people and animals respond to stressful situations. In order to survive, ancient man (even modern man) had to be able to respond instantly and appropriately to any challenging situation. Through a system in which the brain recognizes danger, hormones instantaneously are secreted into the blood stream and speed their way to the various parts of the body preparing it for flight or for fight. One of the essential stimulating substances is *adrenalin*. If no reaction occurs, i.e., if your body has been stimulated to react, yet does not respond in a physical way, the adrenalin persists in your system and in a sense keeps your muscles in a "heightened state of activity," which causes your muscles to stay tense and tight.

For better or worse this ancient "alarm system" persists in all of us. For better, it still protects you and helps you survive in an ever-increasingly complex world. For worst, it constantly produces a state of "body alert" to which we do not respond physically and which leads to fatigue and tension in muscles. The adrenalin in your system increases your heart rate, makes you breathe faster, elevates your blood pressure, closes the little vessels in your hands and feet so that the muscles can have more oxygen bearing blood, and tightens or tenses up all your muscles. Fortunately, you don't have to worry about dinosaurs devouring you, but you are still stressed continually in life and often are unable to react appropriately. Driving in your car and escaping a serious accident leaves you with your heart pounding in your mouth and your hands trembling. As the adrenalin effect dissipates, the anxiety is relieved, and your system returns to normal. But meanwhile you have experienced a real "alarm reaction."

Stress and tension are not selective. They spare no one. The man with a million dollars will be just as anxious about keeping and making more as the man with empty pockets is anxious about where his next meal is coming from. And if their respective anxieties remain unresolved, both are likely to have back pain as a result.

Psychosomatic Back Pain

I was going to say at the beginning of this chapter that I was embarking on it with a certain amount of ambivalence. My ambivalence relates to the whole question of psychosomatic back pain—the kind of pain that is often described as "all in your mind"—in other words, back pain that has no causes in the back or anywhere else in the body for that matter.

The pain that comes from emotional stress and tension is certainly not imaginary. Yet my experience indicates that all too often doctors are inclined to dismiss certain conditions associated with back pain as "all in the mind." If they can't find definite physical symptoms they will tell their patients there's nothing wrong and send them home.

Now stress, tension and emotional fatigue, as you have

seen, all can lead to back pain. But there's another psychological cause of back pain which, though unreal according to our
clinical criteria, is still very real to the people who suffer it, in
spite of the fact that it may be mind-induced.

Some people make more of their back pain than others.
This is due in part, perhaps, to the fact that some have lower
thresholds of pain than others. It can also be due to efforts
to obtain attention. Children have attention-getting devices,
but we amusedly forgive these because they are children and
we feel we understand them. Adults have attention-getting
devices too, but of these we are not so forgiving. We tend to
dismiss such adults as childish and have nothing more to do
with them if we can help it.

I think this is a mistake. I've said earlier that the ideal doctor treats not only the pain, but the patient. There are many
people in this world who do have "imaginary" back pain. At
least it's imaginary to everyone who looks for its clinical
causes and comes up with nothing. But to the patient it's not
imaginary. It's real, whatever the psychological reasons may
be.

But psychosomatic pain can be a tricky business; thus my
ambivalence. For a long time I thought it proper and necessary to treat psychosomatic cases of back pain by attacking
the real cause—the psychological aberrations behind it. This
usually meant referral to a psychiatrist in the hopes that he
could solve the patient's problem. But a recent experience
has forced me to review my previous conviction.

I treated a young man who was admitted to the hospital
with a diagnosis of slipped disc. The patient had severe pain
in his lower back with sciatic radiation into his leg—certainly
the classic signs of such a disorder. He had had two previous
episodes of back pain, neither of which had required hospitalization.

It was routine in the hospital I was attached to at the time
for all patients admitted with diagnosed disc problems to be
examined by a neurologist. After the neurologist had completed his evaluation he informed me that he was convinced
that the young man did not have a slipped disc, indeed, that
he did not even have a back problem. He was familiar with
the patient's history and was convinced that the young man
had reached an emotional situation at home with which he
was unable to cope. His escape, the neurologist assured me,
was to develop psycho-spontaneous back pain so that he

would become incapacitated and avoid having to face his problems.

After looking at all the diagnostic results I agreed that the young man did not have a disc problem and deferred to the neurologist, who took over the case. He went on to treat the patient with psychotherapy, and eventually the young man's pain subsided. He left the hospital without back pain and with the knowledge, as a result of his therapy, that the cause of his pain was emotional.

About a year later I was called to see a woman patient on the psychiatric floor of the hospital who had fallen and broken her hip. As I walked down the corridor toward her ward I was surprised to encounter the young man with the psychosomatic slipped disc. I tried to speak to him. Not only did he not recognize me, he was also unaware of where he was. He was in a complete schizophrenic state.

When I talked to the neurologist about him later that day, he explained to me that the young man had come up against a situation which had crushed him emotionally. Since he had learned and accepted that all his previous episodes of back pain were psychologically induced, he could no longer use this as a crutch to escape from his problems. The pressure of his most recent emotional episode had been so great that his psyche could not cope with it. No longer having the relief valve of back pain, he broke down completely and had to be rushed to the psychiatric department of the hospital.

I relate this true story to give you an idea of the trickiness of psychosomatic pain. Sometimes, it would seem, it does not pay to take people's crutches away from them. The young man might have been able to get through life with an occasional backache now and then. But then again, who knows?

The lesson I learned is that when you take one crutch away from a patient you must support him with another. The poor fellow who had his back pain taken away from him should have had continued psychotherapy until he developed enough emotional stability to stand on his own feet without support.

Part III

The Control of Back Pain

18.

So You Want to Beat Your Back Pain

People who suffer from back problems are unusually prone to try all sorts of fast cures or to accept the advice of their friends or to send away for some special item which will be their panacea. Hundreds of fads regarding back pain come and go. Unfortunately, there are individuals who seek profit from the miseries of others, who subsequently take advantage of the anxiety and ignorance of all too many back sufferers. Because 90 percent of back pain subsides without any treatment, the relief of pain is often attributed to the device or method used. Therefore, these fads or devices gain credibility. The key, the essential factor and treatment of back pain, is not simply getting rid of the pain itself, but to prevent the pain from recurring and to restore the individual to a normal functioning life. The gimmicks and fads *cannot* do this. Your back suffering can only be relieved and prevented by strengthening the muscles that support your spine and by stretching the contracted muscles that strain your spine. The concept is logical, simple, not difficult to perform, and it works.

Another reason fads and gimmicks have done so well in the past is because our modern society has conditioned us to expect the quick and easy answer to everything. If we can travel to Europe in six hours when a hundred years ago it took six weeks; if we can watch a battle unfolding in a South Vietnam rice paddy a few hours after it's happened when a hundred years ago it would have taken a month or more to even learn that the battle had occurred; if we can ask someone halfway across the world a question and receive an immediate answer when a hundred years ago the whole process would have taken months—then why not an instant cure for back pain?

Modern life has many virtues, not the least of which is the comparative ease and rapidity with which we are able to get things done, using the up-to-date tools and aids we have at our disposal. One of the drawbacks to this, however, is that we expect that we should be able to get *all* things done quickly and easily, including the overcoming of chronic back pain. This, of course, is not so. Yet many of us are slow to realize it, which accounts for the fact that the quacks are still successfully promoting the "quick" and "magic" cure for your back.

When All Is Said and Done

When all is said and done, the control and riddance of your back pain is up to you.

A psychiatrist once told me that it did not matter to him how many insights a patient achieved in his office. What he cared about was the work a patient did on his own away from the doctor—how the patient applied his newly gained insights to the unhappy state of his life.

The same goes for back pain victims. If you suffer from back pain you can only be led, like the proverbial horse to water, to therapy; the doctor cannot force you to drink. The burden is on you to help yourself—not on quacks, not on pseudo-legitimate practitioners of vaguely understood healing "arts," not on licensed manipulators or masseurs, not even on medical specialists.

Almost invariably, the conquest of back pain requires home treatment that should be prescribed and supervised by a doctor but must be carried out by the patient on his own. This is the key concept of ideal back-pain therapy. I have almost never seen a back-pain sufferer whom I could not help in some manner. Mind you, sufferers who seek early treatment will invariably fare better than those who put it off. In many cases of back pain, especially the organic diseases I've acquainted you with, there is no cure, but no matter how long the disease has lasted or how severe it has become, something can be done to help. Effective preventive and restorative therapy has always been available for back-pain victims in the form of therapeutic exercise.

But many sufferers expect too much too soon. They cherish the misconception that merely seeing a doctor will immediately solve their problems, that the doctor will do something mysterious *to* or *for* them that will send them away pain-free and cured.

In ideal back-pain treatment a doctor does something quite simple *with* a patient, not to or for him. He helps the patient get started—with a correct diagnosis, with immediate pain relieving drugs, and with an individualized home-therapy program. The doctor then helps the patient to keep going, altering the treatment when necessary.

But the results depend ultimately on what the patient does himself. Having been properly motivated to begin therapy, a patient also needs to become as well informed about the causes, nature and consequences of his problem as he would be about other areas of his life—business, hobbies, children. There is no substitute for really knowing the facts. That is why everyone who suffers from back pain should see a doctor and get a correct diagnosis and a proper therapeutic regimen. The more knowledgeable and sophisticated a backache sufferer is about his affliction and its treatment, the more he will achieve in his attempts to overcome it. In ideal back-pain treatment, then, the patient is an active participant, not a passive, submissive object of treatment. And it is the patient who determines whether the treatment will succeed or fail.

Your Attitude Toward Your Back Pain

I was really frustrated the other day when a woman patient of mine came in and complained that her back pain kept returning. She told me that when her back gets bad she lies down on the floor and does her exercises. After a week or so of exercise her pain vanishes and she feels great again. Then she discontinues her exercises until the next bout of pain occurs. Her complaint was not so much about her backache as about the fact that her backache was recurring with more frequency.

And no wonder. This lady has a poor attitude towards her back. She thinks that sporadic exercise is all she needs. She is wrong. She has been shown repeatedly through her personal experience how exercise can relieve her back pain. What she's simply not able to get into her head is the fact that her exercises are not only designed to relieve her pain when it occurs, they are designed to prevent the pain from occurring altogether. If this lady would take the trouble to learn something about her back and why its pain recurs, she would be more likely to understand the mechanics of her back problem and get it under control for good.

My most successful patients have taught me the most important lesson I have learned as a specialist in back problems —that it is not enough to treat a problem; one must help to educate and motivate the person with the problem.

My friend Shakespeare wrote in *The Merchant of Venice*, "What wouldst thou have, a serpent sting thee twice?" Apparently many people wouldst.

By now you should have a pretty good understanding of the anatomy and mechanics of your back. You should be well aware of all the possible causes of back pain. You should be on the way to being convinced that your back pain can be controlled and eventually put to rest through good posture and regular exercises, both of which enable you to improve the alignment of your spine and to strengthen its supporting muscles.

As you know, the majority of back problems are due to poor posture and to weak musculature. The continued presence of these insufficiencies often leads to degenerative disc disease, early osteoarthritis, and other serious disorders. You've learned that back pain and disability are a result of several factors working together—poor posture, weak musculature, emotional and physical fatigue; plus, perhaps, traumatic factors, defects, infections, hormonal changes, pregnancy and the aging process. In other words, *your back pain is most likely the result of a combination of factors*. But whether you have simple chronic strain or an incurable back disease, exercise can help you to control and possibly eliminate your pain.

A word of caution. It is not my intention in this book to make a doctor or diagnostician out of you. If you try to diagnose and treat yourself, "you have a fool for a patient." If you have back pain, you should have it diagnosed by a trained and experienced professional.

What I am trying to do in this book is give you an understanding of your back and its potential problems so that you will be emotionally and intellectually better motivated to conquer the pain they cause you.

Whenever a patient of mine "moves"—that is, reacts to his or her back pain as if fighting off a murderous attacker—I feel at ease because I know that this patient will do well, no matter how severe or complex the causes of his pain may be. I have also learned that patients who are uneducated about their back pain and its causes will be unmotivated and uncooperative in their therapy, and will usually fare badly, even when their pain is mild.

Your choice is obvious. Learning about the problem you have, learning about the problems you could develop if the present problem is ignored, learning what needs to be done and what to expect, all provide important truths. These truths make you free to act on your problem in the correct manner. And act you better, for if you do not the consequences may be severe.

If you think I'm trying to frighten you unnecessarily, then come spend a day with me in my hospital. Too many back-pain victims do not see a doctor and fail to get to work on rebuilding their backs until they are on the point of becoming disabled. A recent article in the *Wall Street Journal* pointed out that "many persons are needlessly stoical in the face of the discomfort of backache, while others hop from specialist to specialist seeking the magic cure." The second part of this article describes the other mistake many people make. They join the treatment treadmill, which in its way is just as bad as ignoring your back pain, because it indicates that they are equally inclined to avoid the responsibility of solving their back problems by themselves.

No doctor can cure back pain in his office. He can alleviate the pain—he can relieve it, lessen it, diminish it or modify it. He cannot cure it. The only one who can cure it is you.

The Importance of the Muscles

Most of you take good health and strong muscles for granted, especially when you are young or in the prime of your life. However, an illness or the inability to walk up a flight of steps chastens you and quickly changes your attitude. Because muscles are hidden under the skin, you tend to ignore them. You forget that without your muscles you cannot speak, cannot walk, cannot wash your face, and cannot even hold a baby in your arms. Some muscles, such as those comprising the stomach, intestines, and heart, work independently of conscious control; but the muscles that allow us to be mobile and active are under direct control. One of the worse tragedies that I see is the person who has sustained an injury to his neck that permanently damages the spinal cord causing paralysis of both arms and legs. Nothing so dramatically demonstrates the importance of muscles.

In addition to the obvious activity of muscles in moving limbs and supporting the spine, your muscles also play a significant role in overall well-being. Muscles in the arms and legs massage blood vessels and aid circulation. The stimulation of activity improves digestion and intestinal function. And of course, general exercise helps to reduce tension and stress.

The voluntary muscles, those that you can control, are strengthened by use and will atrophy or weaken with disuse. In other words, "You lose it if you don't use it."

Every teenager who becomes body conscious is aware that exercises will not only strengthen muscles but will improve the appearance of the body. You know that in order to have strong muscles, exercise is essential. Muscles have to be used in order to be strengthened and built up. The athlete who competes for a marathon slowly strengthens his muscles and endurance, but he must train regularly as well as vigorously in order to achieve his goal. No one in their right mind would try to run a marathon without proper training. Yet, in a sense, we are all in a marathon, all of us running through life, and most of us do not train properly. We do not strengthen our bodies and improve our endurance. We neglect our back muscles so that they cannot withstand the stress and strain of keeping our bodies upright as we take that long run through life. If you want a healthy back, you must have healthy and strong muscles, and you are the only one who can achieve that goal for yourself.

How do you neglect or abuse your back muscles? You do it first through sloppy posture. Then through inactivity. Remember, a blacksmith's arm is strong because he uses it. And what makes it strong are its muscles. When your back muscles become weak through poor posture and lack of exercise, and when they become tense and overstressed through emotional and physical fatigue and irritation, they cannot do their share in keeping your back erect. Consequently too much strain falls on the bones and ligaments of your spine.

Now, we abuse or neglect our back muscles every day in uncountable ways—that's a fact of life. I'm not so interested in having you change your way of life and your manner of earning a living—for instance, I don't suggest you all go out and become blacksmiths—as I am in having you understand how to counteract the effects your way of life has on your back. And the only way to counteract them is to be conscious every day of your back and pursue the kind of beneficial exercises that will enable you to control these effects and avoid pain.

Remember, once you've developed a back problem, it is never really cured. But it can get well. And it can stay well. If you want to have a healthy and properly functioning back, without disability and without pain, and without the feeling that you're going to be "walking on eggs" for the rest of your life, you have to work for it. You must discipline yourself to do the simple back-strengthening exercises which I am going to set out in the next chapter, and to stand, sit and bend in the right ways. You must continue this program for the rest of your life. Whether your back pain is major or minor, start now! Don't wait until it develops into something worse.

Okay, enough preaching. The proof is in the pudding, so let's get on with the exercise program.

19.

The Therapeutic Exercise Program

Therapeutic exercise is the least appreciated but the most important part of treatment for chronic and recurring back pain. Unfortunately, those who have back pain must be their own training coaches. If they want to get rid of their back pain they must faithfully do prescribed exercises. Most people hate to exercise, and this is why its benefits are so poorly valued. But exercise may often make the difference between leading an active, pain-free life and being contorted and disabled. Those people who overcome their natural antipathy to exercise soon become devoted converts.

Unless your back problem came about directly as a result of some sudden severe injury or of an organic disease, your condition is probably the consequence of four factors: habitual poor posture, chronic strain, weakened back muscles, and the stress-tension-fatigue syndrome. Taken together these four factors constitute the major single cause of back instability and its subsequent pain and disability. The most significant component of this four-in-one cause are your back muscles, because when the muscles break down, your back breaks down. In order to return your back to some semblance of its normal self, you must return your muscles to normal.

Because an exercise program in the past has failed to improve your back problems, it should not discourage you from trying again. Too often exercises are given without proper instructions in performing them, or in their respective goals. The cursory instructions "here are the exercises, do them every day and your back shall get better" are totally inadequate. As I told you earlier in this book, I have my own back problems, and I have experimented with hundreds of back exercises. I personally know how difficult some of them are, and how difficult it is to explain specific goals for each. Furthermore, exercises should be grouped according to specific purposes. So, if in the past you had not been educated in your exercise program, it almost certainly would have been doomed to fail.

The exercises that follow in this chapter are those I have found to be most effective for strengthening and maintaining a healthy back. They have evolved through my own back experiences and through care of thousands of back patients. The exercises are not strenuous, are easy to perform, and require no special equipment, except for self-discipline. They are limited in number because I have discovered that when I prescribe many exercises for my patients, the exercises often do not get done. You may already be familiar with some of these exercises in one form or another, because today none of the back exercises are original nor is there only one exercise that is sufficient to strengthen the back.

Although 85 percent of patients with back problems can do these exercises without harm and thus control their back pain, certain cautions are important.

1. If your pain is severe or associated with sciatica, you should consult your doctor before you begin the exercises to make certain that they are appropriate for you.

2. Do not begin the exercises until the pain has subsided. If your muscles are in spasm, exercise may aggravate them.

3. If the exercises, at any time, increase your pain, consult your doctor before resuming or continuing them.

With these cautions observed, four basic rules must be followed diligently.

1. Initially, until you have sufficiently strengthened your supporting muscles, the exercises should be done twice a day. This generally requires three months of twice-a-day exercises, and afterward maintenance can be on a daily basis. I prefer to do my exercises first thing in the morning before breakfast or shower.

2. Begin the exercises slowly. Do not strain or become overeager to progress. Make certain you are able to do each exercise well and easily before you increase the number of repititions or proceed to the next exercise.

3. When you first begin the exercises, have someone observe you perform them and read aloud the description of each exercise. This prevents you from doing the exercises improperly, which could limit the benefits you get from the exercises or even cause additional distress and discomfort.

4. Finally, firmly burn into your mind that the exercise program is for *now* and *always*. It becomes boring, but so does brushing your teeth.

As busy as you are, you will find that the time spent on your exercises (about twenty minutes) rewards you with being able to lead an active, painless-back life.

The Eight General Exercises

I have separated the exercises into two sections. The first consists of eight general exercises which all sufferers of back pain can profitably do without putting excess stresses on their backs. These exercises are designed to eliminate lower-back pain. Whether you suffer from mild pain due to chronic fatigue or severe pain due to structural instability, you can do these exercises without fear of harming yourself. Indeed, not only will you not harm yourself if you do them according to instructions, you will help yourself. The second section consists of three exercises for specific upper back and neck pain and two for relief of pain due to the excessive dorsal kyphosis or rounded back brought about by Scheuermann's Disease in young people.

The eight general lower-back exercises have been proven over the years to be the best exercises for improving spinal joint mobility and strengthening the guy-wire system of the spine. They are not intended to make a muscle-man or muscle-woman out of you.

All the exercises should be done on a firm surface, preferably a carpeted floor. They should all be done slowly and carefully, with a minimum of straining. Usually it takes three weeks before you are comfortable doing them, but by that time you will have begun to notice definite positive results.

I have further divided the eight general exercises into two sets of four each. The first set consists of stretching and loosening exercises of the deeper muscles and other structures around your spine; the second set consists of muscle-strength ening exercises. You should start off with the first four exercises alone. Once you have mastered these and have become comfortable with them—after two or three weeks, say—*you should then proceed to add, one at a time, the second four exercises.*

Remember that when you start the program you should do the exercises twice daily—morning and night. With the exception of the last of the eight exercises, the standard starting position is lying flat on your back with your knees bent and raised, soles of your feet on the floor, and your hands and arms flat out by your side for easy balance. This position is very important. By raising your knees and having your back flat against the floor, you relax all the stress and strain on your hamstring, abdominal and lower-back muscles, as well as on your sciatic nerve. You also reduce your lumbar spinal curve.

Each exercise should be repeated five times in its entirety at the beginning. All should be done slowly, carefully and deliberately, with concentration and close attention to correct technique. *Do not run through them just to get them over with.* Gradually, as they become easier to do, you can add additional repetitions until you are able to accomplish ten of them without excessive strain. Once you have this capability, you will then be ready to go on a once-a-day maintenance program.

Exercise 1. (Figure 15.)

KNEE-TO-CHEST RAISE. *Step A*. From the standard starting position, pull your left knee to your chest as far as it will go without causing you pain. Hold, count slowly to five, then return your leg to the starting position.

Step B. Repeat the same maneuver with your right leg, drawing your right knee as close as you can to your chest, holding it there for a count of five, then returning your leg to the starting position.

Step C. Now bring both knees up toward your chest, allowing them to separate slightly so that they point toward your shoulders. When knees are as close to chest as you can get them, hold for a count of five, then slowly return legs to starting position.

Run through this exercise five times to begin with, doing all three parts each time. Once you can do the entire exercise five times without difficulty, gradually increase the repetitions to ten. Do not use your arms or hands to help you in raising your knees—they are only for balance, and if you use them for leverage you will dilute the therapeutic value of the exercise. Likewise, do not strain or lunge—do the maneuvers slowly and deliberately, and always be in control of those parts of your body you are moving from one position to another.

The purpose of this exercise is to stretch out the stiff and tightened muscles, ligaments and joints of your lower back.

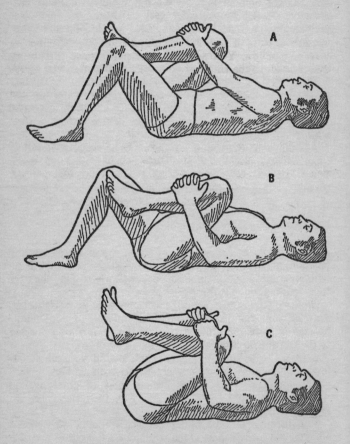

FIG. 15   Exercise 1: Knee-to-chest raise.

You will find after awhile that it is very useful in relieving the constant feeling of strain and fatigue you have there.

Exercise 2. (Figure 16.)

PELVIC TILT. In this exercise you simply contract your buttocks muscles while lying in the standard starting position. Hold your buttocks clenched for a count of five, then relax them, all the time keeping your lower spine flattened against the floor. Do not try to flatten your spine by using your legs or abdominal muscles; rather, do it by concentrating on tightening the mucles of your buttocks, squeezing them together as hard as you can. You will feel your pelvis raise slightly as you do so, and the small of your back will flatten out by itself.

The purpose of this exercise is to strengthen your gluteus maximus muscles, which, when in good condition, prevent excessive lumbar spinal curve (swayback) and reduce fatigue when you stand for long periods of time.

Again, do the exercise five times to begin with, contracting your buttocks slowly and as tightly as you can. Hold them firmly clenched for a count of five each time, with a brief

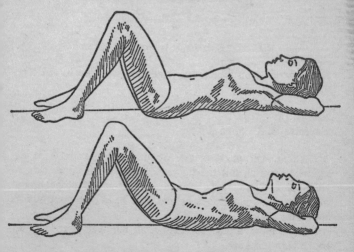

FIG. 16   Exercise 2: Pelvic tilt.

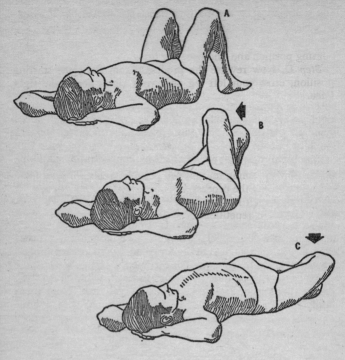

FIG. 17   Exercise 3: Lateral trunk stretch.

rest between each repetition. Gradually work up to ten repetitions.

Exercise 3. (Figure 17.)

LATERAL TRUNK STRETCH. *Step A.* This exercise is designed to stretch out the tightened muscles on either side of your spine. Start in the standard knees-raised position, but this time place your hands behind your head with your elbows flat on the floor.

Step B. Now, cross your bent right leg over your left, just above your left knee.

Step C. Using the weight of your right leg to force your

left knee, press your left knee to the right as far as possible, preferably so that your left knee touches the floor. Hold your left knee to the floor for a count of five, then return it to the starting position and uncross your legs.

Step D. Now reverse the process. From the same starting position, cross your left leg over your right, above the right knee.

Step E. Using the weight of your left leg as it's crossed over the right, force your right knee to the left until it touches the floor or comes as close to it as possible. Hold there for a count of five.

Step F. Return to the starting position, uncross your legs and, still maintaining the starting position, relax for a moment before repeating the process.

Alternate each leg five times to begin with and work gradually up to ten repetitions for each side. Again, do the exercise slowly and deliberately, without any cheating or short-cutting. If you are at first unable to get either or both knees to the floor without excessive strain on your back and limbs, try to get them as close to the floor as possible and keep working at it until you are able to touch the floor with your knees. At all times keep your upper back flat on the floor, using your elbows to achieve this balance. As you master this very valuable exercise you will feel the muscles in either side of your torso stretch with each alternating maneuver.

Exercise 4. (Figure 18.)

SINGLE STRAIGHT-LEG RAISE. *Step A.* From the standard starting position, straighten out your left leg and press it flat against the floor with your left knee rigid. Then, as slowly as you can, and without using your hands and arms for leverage, raise the straightened leg as high as you can, until you get pain or excessive tightness in your thigh. When you've raised the leg as high as you can, hold for a count of five. Then, still as slowly and deliberately as you can, let your leg drop back to the floor, still keeping your knee straight. Relax for a moment, then repeat for a total of five consecutive repetitions.

Step B. When your left leg is back on the floor after the last repetition, return to the standard starting position. Then straighten out your right leg and repeat the exercise, slowly raising your straightened leg as high as you can, holding for a count of five, and slowly returning it to the floor. Again, repeat for a total of five consecutive repetitions.

When doing this exercise never swing your legs up and do not use your hands to help you push. Keep your lower back flat on the floor as you raise each straightened leg, and constantly strive to raise each leg as high as you can, working

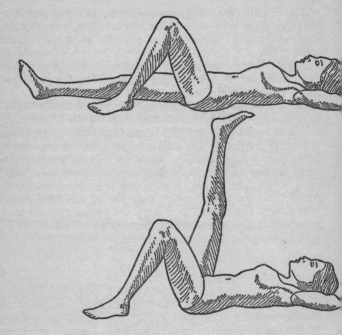

FIG. 18   Exercise 4: Single straight-leg raise.

gradually, over a period of time, up to ten consecutive repetitions for each leg.

This is another valuable exercise for stretching and strengthening your tight hamstring, buttocks and hip muscles, which go a long way toward preserving and supporting your lower back.

After you have mastered the first four exercises and can do each of them ten times comfortably, you are ready to go on to the second set of four, which begin with Exercise 5. Whereas the first four are designed mainly to aid you in *stretching out* the supporting structures of your back, the second four are designed to *strengthen* the important muscles that keep your spine in proper balance and configuration.

Exercise 5. (Figure 19.)

HALF SIT-UPS. *Step A*. Again, starting from the standard position, slowly raise your head and neck until your chin touches the top of your chest.

Step B. As you maintain this position, and without raising your mid- or lower back off the floor, reach both hands forward and place them on the tops of both your knees, which are bent. Hold this position for a count of five.

Step C. After you've counted to five, slowly return to the starting position, relax for a moment, then repeat.

This exercise, like the others, should be done five times to begin with and gradually increased to ten repetitions. It strengthens your abdominal and lower-back muscles, doing the work of conventional sit-ups without causing the back strain conventional sit-ups often produce. As with all the other exercises in this program, it is important that it be done slow-

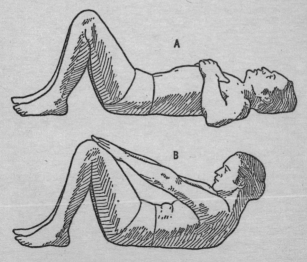

FIG. 19   Exercise 5: Half sit-ups.

ly, deliberately and with concentration. As your abdominal muscles become strengthened, they will better be able to provide the frontal support your back requires, the lack of which is so often a contributing factor in back pain.

Exercise 6. (Figure 20.)

NOSE-TO-KNEE TOUCH. *Step A.* From the standard starting position, bring your left knee slowly to your chest, as in Exercise 1. As you clasp it tightly against your chest with both hands, extend and straighten your right leg until it is flat on the floor.

Step B. Keeping your lower back flat on the floor, raise your head and bring it forward until you can touch your nose to your bent knee. Hold your nose against your knee for a count of five.

Step C. Slowly drop your head back to the floor. Relax for a moment, still keeping your left knee clamped to your chest, then raise your head and touch your nose to your knee again.

Do this exercise five times with your left knee raised to your chest, then switch and do it five times with your right

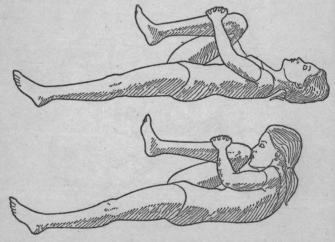

FIG. 20   Exercise 6: Nose-to-knee touch.

knee raised. This exercise strengthens your abdominal muscles and at the same time stretches the opposite hip flexors.

Exercise 7. (Figure 21.)

SCISSORS. *Step A.* This is a standard exercise used in most calisthentic programs for the abdominal, hip and back muscles. I would like you to do it this way. Start again from the standard position, bring both knees to your chest, and hold there for a moment while you concentrate on keeping good balance with your back flat on the floor.

Step B. Using your hands to balance yourself, straighten both legs into the air together.

Step C. With your legs straight and extended vertically, very slowly scissor them front-to-back ten times, opening the scissors as wide as you can each time while maintaining good control and balance.

Step D. Once you've completed the front-to-back scissor, proceed to scissor your legs laterally or crossways ten

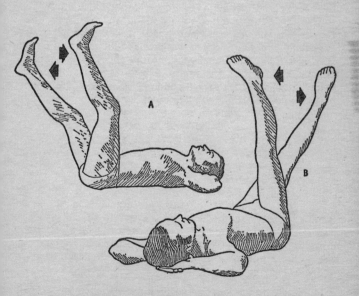

FIG. 21   Exercise 7: Scissors.

more times, alternating right leg *over* left, right leg *under* left.

Step E. On the completion of the lateral scissors, slowly return to the starting position, first by slowly bringing your knees down to your chest, then by returning your feet to the floor.

Relax for a few moments, then repeat the exercise again. This exercise will further stretch out and strengthen your hamstring, lower-back and hip muscles, and will also strengthen your abdominal muscles.

Exercise 8. (Figure 22.)

HIP HYPEREXTENSION. *Step A.* For this exercise you turn over onto your stomach. Lie flat and let your hands and arms fall naturally over your shoulders.

Step B. Stiffen your left leg, making sure your knee is as rigid as you can make it, then slowly raise your stiffened leg from the hip. Do not rotate your pelvis in order to get your leg off the floor—keep it flat. Raise and lower your left leg five times consecutively.

Step C. Return to the starting position, relax for a moment, then stiffen your right leg and repeat the exercise five times.

Initially you may find it very difficult to lift your legs off the floor at all. Do not despair, and do not cheat, it will come if you work at it. If all you are able to do at first is tighten up your buttocks and leg muscles and get your leg off just slightly, that's fine. Starting with five repetitions for each leg, work up to ten. When you are able to lift each leg between ten and fifteen degrees off the floor ten consecutive times without undue strain, you will have reached your goal for this exercise. The exercise stretches and strengthens your hip muscles and at the same time further strengthens your buttocks and lower-back muscles.

In doing Exercises 5 through 8 you should start with 5, do it for a few days until it becomes comfortable, then add 6. Do 6 for a few days, then add 7, and finally 8. It should take you between two and three weeks before you are doing all eight exercises. Stick with your twice-a-day schedule for another two to three weeks, or until you have mastered each exercise and your back pain has subsided.

Once this occurs you can go on a maintenance schedule of once a day, but keep to that schedule faithfully. Don't think

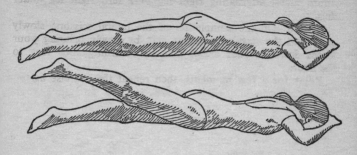

FIG. 22   Exercise 8: Hip hyperextension.

that once your pain and stiffness have subsided you can do without the exercises. If you continue to do them you will then be able to go out and resume your normal physical activities—even certain sports—without fear of your back pain recurring. If you stop doing them, your back pain will sooner or later return, and you'll be back where you started.

I have deliberately kept this therapeutic exercise program limited to eight exercises. I have found from experience when you give too many exercises, none of them get done. This combination of exercises has proved to be the most successful with my patients, and it takes no more than fifteen to twenty minutes a day to accomplish it. It is certainly worth it to devote this small amount of time to ensuring yourself a healthy back free of pain and instability.

I have done these exercises myself for the past eight years. They have proved a great success for me and they have proved a great success for my patients. I am sure they will prove a great success for you.

If your back instability is mild when you begin this program, it certainly wouldn't hurt you to add a few conventional calisthenic exercises to your regimen after you finish the special therapeutic maneuvers. Being a former athlete, I wind up my daily session with ten or twelve push-ups to keep my upper body muscles in good tone.

Three Special Exercises

Obviously we cannot divorce the neck from the rest of the spine. Many people suffer from pain in the upper back

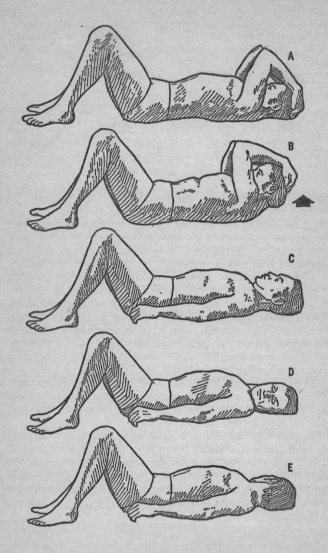

FIG. 23   Exercise 1: Neck stretch.

and neck. Most pain of this sort is due to poor posture and the accompanying stresses it places on the muscles of the region. Some of it is also due to disc degeneration associated with arthritis, trauma, or aging. No matter the cause, there are therapeutic exercises that will relieve the pain. I will present here the three most effective ones.

Exercise 1. (Figure 23.)

THE NECK STRETCH. *Steps A and B.* Once again, begin in the standard starting position for the lower-back exercises —flat on your back on the floor with your knees raised. Place the palms of your hands against the back of your head. Holding your elbows together, bring your chin towards your chest.

Step C. Using your hands to press your head forward, force your chin back off your chest for a count of five, still exerting pressure from the rear so that your chin does not move.

Steps D and E. Rotate your head twice to either side, keeping your chin as tightly to your chest as you can and trying to touch your shoulders with it.

Repeat this sequence five times and work gradually up to ten repetitions. This exercise is a difficult one. At first you may experience a grinding or cracking sensation, but you can safely ignore this; you may also find that it makes you a bit dizzy, but keep at it. Once you are able to stretch out the tensed and tightened structures of your neck you will find that a lot of the stiffness and pain you are experiencing will disappear.

Exercise 2. (Figure 24.)

SHOULDER BLADE PINCH. *Step A.* This exercise is specifically designed for those of you who have weak shoulder and upper-back muscles. It works wonders for stenographers, accountants, writers and others who have to spend long periods sitting at desks or typewriters. Begin in the standard starting position, but with your hands clasped behind your head and your elbows flat against the floor. Then try to draw your shoulder blades together, elevating your chest off the floor.

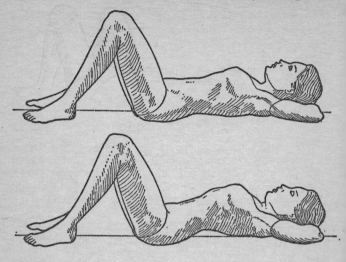

FIG. 24   Exercise 2: Shoulder blade pinch.

Step B. When you get your shoulder blades as close together as you can, hold them there for a count of three, then relax. Repeat the exercise five times to begin with and gradually work up to ten repetitions.

Exercise 3. (Figure 25.)

THE ARM STRETCH. *Step 1.* Again from the standard starting position, bring your left arm over your head and stretch it as far as you can to the rear, leaving your right arm on the floor beside your hip.

Step 2. Take a deep breath, then stretch the two arms away from each other as far as you can, your left arm reaching for the wall above your head, your right arm reaching for your toes. Hold the stretch for a count of three, then relax and begin again.

Do this exercise ten times with your left arm over your head, then switch your arms and do it ten more times with your right arm over your head. This will stretch and strengthen the tight muscles of your upper back and will also improve the range of motion in your shoulders.

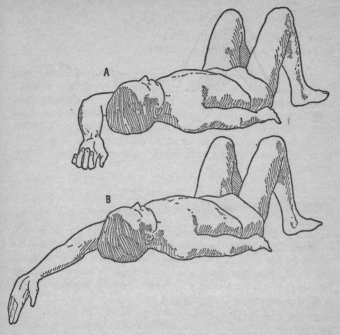

FIG. 25   Exercise 3: Arm stretch.

Exercises for the Elderly or Infirm

If you are elderly or infirm, you must be a little more careful in your approach to these back exercises. You are the best judge of how much you can take on. If you find this complete program a bit too strenuous, do not despair. You can still do some of the exercises and gain great benefits from them.

I suggest limiting the exercises you do at the beginning to numbers 1, 2, and 4 of the general exercise program. These are perfectly safe for you, and once you have mastered them, you can proceed to the other exercises of the general program, eliminating Exercise 8. If in addition you have neck and upper-back pain, I would recommend that you skip Exercise 1 of the special program—the Neck Stretch—and do only Exercises 2 and 3, which should not be too strenuous for you.

Two Exercises for Pain from Excessive Round-Shoulderedness

Many young people have excessive round-shouldered posture, caused by poor postural habits or by Scheuermann's Disease. In either case they are likely to have upper- and mid-back pain. If they expect control and relief of their pain they must improve their posture and strengthen their shoulder and upper-back muscles at as early an age as possible. Here are two exercises which will go a long way to achieving these goals.

Exercise 1. (Figure 26.)

BACK ARCH. The young person should lie on the floor with a small, firm pillow beneath his waist. He should place his hands by his sides and then raise his neck and upper back off the floor, holding his upper body arched for a count of five. He should then relax and repeat it again. He should start with five repetitions, raising and arching his back as high as he comfortably can, and gradually build up to ten. This exercise will strengthen the entire extensor muscles of the spine. As these grow stronger, they will take some of the loads and stresses off the spinal column and help relieve the pain.

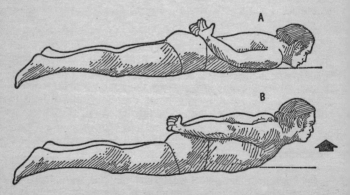

FIG. 26   Exercise 1: Back arch, two stages.

Exercise 2. (Figure 27.)

NECK-AND-SHOULDER ARCH: This exercise is started from the same position as the back arch, except the hands should be clasped behind the neck and elbows against the floor. The young person should then slowly raise his neck and elbows as high off the floor as he or she can, keeping the rest of the body pressed to the floor. The raised position should be held for a count of five, then slowly relaxed. After a short rest the exercise should be repeated. Start with five repetitions

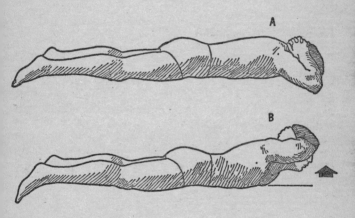

FIG. 27   Exercise 2: Neck-and-shoulder arch.

and work up to ten, as in the Back Arch. This exercise strengthens the muscles of the upper back, shoulders, and neck that have been weakened by the round-shouldered condition; the faithful employment of the exercise will help to relieve the chronic pain caused by the condition.

Summary

I have given you a total of thirteen exercises, eight for the lower back, three for the upper back and neck, and two for Scheuermann's Disease. Do not underrate these exercises because they seem simple and are not numerous. If you are able to perform them in a regular fashion, you will gain control over your back pain and eventually eliminate it.

They are exercises that everyone can do, even people with mild cardiac and respiratory problems. They are not difficult, but they are very effective. Their effect is cumulative—whether your back pain is due to chronic strain or to disc disorder, to postural defects or to arthritis, to systemic disease or to aging, to pregnancy or to emotional fatigue, they will be instrumental in conquering your pain.

But remember, the success of these exercises depends on you, on how willing you are to perform them faithfully and exactly. If you are willing, and you follow it up—well, try them and see.

20.

Advice for Daily Living

The *Wall Street Journal* article to which I alluded in Chapter 18 quotes a suburban Chicago housewife: "I've been walking on eggs since I had my first attack a year ago. I don't think an hour passes without my thinking 'Should I do this? It might be bad for my back.' "

Sound familiar? Most sufferers of chronic back pain spend a good deal of their time fearfully waiting for the next attack to strike. For most, a bad back is a constant source of anxiety, tempering or interfering with just about everything they do. It interferes with their normal physical activities, it practically precludes their participation in their favorite sports and recreation, and it plays havoc with their sex lives.

With proper postural awareness and the faithful performance of our therapeutic exercise regimen, all these factors can be relegated to the ash heap where they belong. With very few exceptions there is no reason why you can't return to your normal activities, to your favorite sports, and to healthy, happy sexual relations. But while you are going through the process of restoring your back to its desirable strength and suppleness and ridding yourself of the pain and anxiety it causes you, you should take some care in how you go about things. Once your pain is gone and your abdominal and back muscles have been restored to good tone and strength, and if you are willing to continue your exercise program, you can then begin to resume most of your normal activities without fear of re-triggering your pain.

Postural Awareness

The back-pain victim, if he is to eliminate his pain, really has to rethink the way he sits, stands and walks. He must constantly counteract the inclination, brought on by the source of his pain, to bend, slouch or stoop. Occasionally I will put a brace on a patient to promote good posture, but most often this is totally unnecessary. Almost immediately patients follow my advice to consciously stand as erect as possible, and to walk and think "tall."

The best means of achieving this is to constantly practice the simple postural exercise I outlined and had you perform in Chapter 8—the one in which you elevate your head as high as you can, at the same time contracting your buttocks so that your pelvis thrusts forward. Again, good posture is not achieved overnight. But it can be achieved—indeed, it must be achieved if you are going to eliminate your back pain. Once achieved, it will go a long way toward preserving your back, and will make the therapeutic exercises that much more effective.

The first step in relieving your back pain is to achieve good posture in all of your body's positions. When standing you must avoid at all times the tendency to stoop, lean over or bend forward or sideways. Should you drop a pencil to the floor, you must bend your knees as you pick it up. You must never lounge in a soft-cushioned armchair, but must sit up straight in a chair with a firm back. At night you should sleep on a firm mattress that has a wooden board underneath. You should use either a small or no pillow for your head, you should not sleep on your stomach, you should always try to keep your knees bent while lying on your side.

The stand-tall postural exercise, plus these postural precautions, will soon have you posture-conscious. Once you've achieved this, it is only a matter of time until good posture becomes second nature to you.

Therapeutic Exercises

I never cease to wonder at the marvels the therapeutic exercises outlined in the last chapter perform. When I first started doing them myself and they worked, I was still a bit cautious in my praise of them—just because they worked for me did not necessarily mean that they would work for everybody. But today, after years of prescribing them for hundreds of other back-pain sufferers, I feel I can safely throw my caution to the winds. They do work for all those who are willing to make them a daily part of their lives.

It is always a thrill for me when a patient breezes into my office a few months after I have prescribed the exercises, especially when the last time I saw him he was hobbling, anxious, fearful, and consumed with pain. The magic transformation can be summed up by five words: *Postural awareness and therapeutic exercise.* Anyone can do it, and at any age.

Like the postural training, the therapeutic exercises are not just cornerstones of back therapy, they must become an intrinsic part of your life. Then and only then will they be able to fulfill their function—to make your back well and give you the freedom from pain and disability you so richly deserve.

Physical Activities

Postural training and therapeutic exercises rebuild your back and rid you of back pain. By themselves, however, they will not necessarily cure the causes of your pain. If you have a collapsed disc, for instance, they can take up much of the stress on your spine created by the disc and therefore relieve the pain, but they will not cause the disc to become uncollapsed. If you suffer from osteoarthritis, for another example, they can again take up some of the stresses and strains on your spine and relieve the pain, but they will not cure the arthritis, although as they strengthen your back they can retard its progression.

Along with the exercises, you must revise some of the major factors in your life which contributed to your problem in the first place. As you've learned, back pain is usually caused by a combination of factors, not the least of which are emotional tension and the fatigue it creates in the structures of your back. Most emotional tension comes from cumulative irritations that fill your life. In other words, it is as though you have an emotional well inside of you that constantly builds up tension and stress. If you can successfully drain off those problems that lead to stress and tension, the

well does not overflow. However, if the stress and tension are
not relieved, the well fills up. And just one more drop, one
insignificant problem, can lead to an overspill of great magnitude. I cannot give you a formula by which to live, or change
your life-style. I can only urge you to examine the little things
that upset you, analyze them and try to place them in proper
prospective, and remember that the anger or distress that you
feel at one moment may be an accumulation of many previous
aggravating incidents.

Inner emotional turmoil produces great tension. Everyone
has problems. Too often these problems are blown out of
proportion and assume a greater magnitude than necessary.
Exercises, as I pointed out before in this book, help to relieve
tension but obviously cannot remove deep-seated anxiety. Often an understanding spouse or a good friend can help by just
listening. However, if the problem persists and becomes disabling, then professional (psychological or psychiatric) help
should be sought.

That, of course, is up to you. But in the meantime you can
avoid many of the bad habits that contribute to muscle fatigue, back pain, stiff neck and nagging headaches. Some of
these habits can be so bad, in fact, that they may lock your
back muscles into set positions for most of the day, thereby
greatly diminishing the effects of your daily exercise program.

Try to start your day in a good mood and remain aloof
from things that would ordinarily irritate you. A bad temper
in the morning will most likely set your mood for the day,
and you'll spend the rest of the day building a skyscraper of
tension on this foundation. At the end of the day you'll find
your back as rigid as a skyscraper, too.

Patients often ask me what constitutes proper dress and
shoes. I believe that it is essential that you wear comfortable
clothes that fit well. Clothes that are too tight restrict body
movements and can interfere with blood circulation. Too
loose-fitting clothes hang on your body and feel uncomfortable. The use of girdles for women has gradually been de-
creasing, and I am pleased by this trend because girdles offer
no back support and do nothing to improve muscle strength.

Proper walking shoes are a must. Narrow tight shoes that
squeeze the feet may look grand but not only are they bad for
your feet, they also prevent normal walking, which can lead
to back strain. High-heeled shoes in particular cause an in-

crease in the sway back posture of the lumbar spine (lordosis) and can be a significant cause of back fatigue, strain and pain.

Sitting is the most strenuous position for your back to maintain for prolonged periods. This is especially true when you have had a history of a bad back. When sitting, your stomach muscles are relaxed, and thus greater stress is placed on your lower back muscles. These muscles fatigue and allow increased strain on the supporting ligaments and intervertebral discs of the lower spine. Therefore, never sit for too long. If your work requires considerable sitting, make certain that you get up every hour or so and walk about, sort of limber up your muscles (it will also help your circulation). Perform the posture exercise described earlier in the book, getting your head up, and taking deep breaths. Swing your arms loosely from your shoulders. Raise them over your head. Raise up on your toes several times to improve the circulation in your legs. If you have been driving, pull over to the edge of the road and get out of the car. Perform these same maneuvers. Let your body relax a bit and then resume your driving. You will find that these exercises, both for sitting at the office or driving a car, will help prevent fatigue and enable you to continue your activity for longer periods.

Physical Activities

Bending and lifting are part of your every day activity. The housewife has to contend with heavy bags of groceries or heavy baskets of wash. The carpenter lifts large, bulky, and often very heavy boards and lumber. The delivery man carries heavy cartons and boxes. The traveler lugs about heavy suitcases and valises. None of these activities may be emotionally stressful, but they certainly can, and do, produce a great deal of physical stress on the body and particularly on the back. There is a right way and a wrong way to lift, whether it be a shoe from the floor or a box of heavy books. Never bend from the waist without first bending the knees. When lifting the object, face it squarely, that is, both feet pointed to the box or carton. Keep the knees bent and lift the object toward your body, then holding it close to your chest and abdomen, slowly straighten your legs and stand erect. When placing that heavy object onto the floor, just reverse the process.

Proper posture when walking or running is, needless to

say, an absolute necessity. So, too, is it an absolute necessity when bending or squatting, reaching or climbing, pushing or pulling. As long as you practice proper posture in your normal physical activities and couple this with your exercises, you will soon be able to accomplish just about anything without fear of straining or re-straining your back and creating new pain or disability.

Sports

For those of you who are athletically inclined, your back pain has probably become a real nemesis and has prevented you from participating in your favorite sports and recreational activities. Indeed, quite often it is participation in these activities that initially triggers back pain and disability. Most orthopaedists can depend on full waiting-rooms of middle-aged executives turned athletes every Monday after the first few nice weekends of spring. The same goes for the fall, when the touch-football fever strikes hundreds of thousands of usually sedentary Frank Merriwells.

Sports activities fall into three categories: team sports, one-on-one contests, and solitary pursuits. Unfortunately the first two usually comprise contests in which there is a good deal of violent twisting and jarring of the back. For someone with either an unhealthy back or an out-of-condition one, such sports should be avoided. The third category, in which the individual can proceed at his or her own pace, is much more salutary to unstable backs.

I would never attempt to discourage an individual from getting as much exercise as he can. Indeed, the more general exercise you can obtain in conjunction with your therapeutic back exercises and within the limitations created by your back problem, the better! However, if you have a proven back instability or weakness, you must approach your favorite sports with good sense.

Swimming is the one sport—and all doctors agree—that is not only *not* harmful to your back but eminently good for it. I encourage all my back patients to make swimming, whenever possible, a regular part of their exercise program. The buoyancy of the water removes the gravitational stresses on your back. The physical motions of swimming exercise all the muscles in your body and are especially beneficial to the back muscles. People with back pain should not try to perform fancy dives off the spring board, of course, but simple, well-executed straight dives are permissible. The best swimming strokes are the overhand crawl and the side stroke. The butterfly stroke should be avoided because it demands a snapping motion of the spine in connection with the double-arm pull.

Long, steady endurance swimming is better than short sprint-type swimming. Sprint swimming tires you out quickly and overstresses your muscles, not giving them enough time to get the good workout they need.

Running is another form of exercise that is extremely beneficial to back-pain sufferers. Many of you will not have water at your disposal for regular swimming, but you can run anywhere. As with swimming, the same general rules apply: long-distance running is better than sprinting because it allows you to give your muscles the full workout they require. Running should be done easily and with good posture, and the distances you run should be built up gradually. The idea is not to exhaust yourself, but to give all the muscles of your body, as well as your heart, lungs and circulatory system, a good workout. It is also important to run on the balls of your feet, not your heels. Naturally, before you start a running program—indeed, before you start any sports and exercise regimen—you should clear it with your doctor.

Skiing is another solitary sport which is permissible. The position in which one skis, if one is skiing properly, is a position which protects the lumbo-sacral spine. I never hesitate to allow an experienced skier who has recovered from his back instability through exercises to resume skiing. However, if you have never skied, I would not advise you to start if you have back problems, because the learning process is drawn out. At the beginning you will find yourself taking spills that could be further injurious to your back.

Yoga exercises and courses have been growing in fashion and popularity in this country for the past few years. In general these exercises are not harmful to the back and in many instances can be beneficial. Yoga exercises are done slowly and deliberately, with a great deal of concentration and thought, all of which is good. I would advise against doing those exercises which cause you to arch your back, however.

Many women have asked me about the advisability of continuing with their ballet or modern dance programs after they've had a back instability develop. In response to this question I consider two factors. One—if they have been dancing for many years and on a regular basis, I feel it is safe for them to continue once they have gained control over their pain and instability by means of the therapeutic exercises. Two—if their back pain is mainly muscular rather than spinal, and they do not have any leg pain, I also feel it is safe to continue. However, in either case, the dance programs must be engaged in regularly so that their bodies, and especially their backs, are used to the rhythms and motions of dance. If they attempt to dance at irregular intervals their movements will not be smooth, and excessive strain on the back muscles will most likely result.

General cosmetic exercise classes are growing in popularity, especially in urban environments. The reason that these classes have become so popular is because people find that they become more faithful when they are in a group exercise situation. Which is fine. Exercising by yourself can get pretty boring after a while, and it is only human to want to measure your progress against that of others. Since many qualified professional exercise instructors are trained physical therapists, or at least have been trained in the principals of physical education, they know what they are doing. Nevertheless, if you are a devotee of such exercise classes, you should inform your instructor that you have had back problems and describe their nature. If he is a good instructor, he will modify your exercises to prevent undue strain on your back and may even give you special exercises that will aid in building up your back muscles.

Beware, however, of dance or exercise instructors who are ready and eager to tell you what's wrong with your back. The dance and exercise business—especially when it involves the cosmetic or "figure-improving" aspects—appeals more to your vanity than it does to your good health. A lot of so-called exercise classes are designed to do nothing more than improve your figure. Which is fine, as far as it goes. But improving your figure is of little use to you if there is not a corresponding improvement in your overall strength, muscle tone and well-being. Quite often you will be urged to go on crash diets or employ "diet pills" or diuretics to help you lose weight. Losing weight, if you are overweight and flabby, is certainly a desirable goal. However, crash diets are often based on low food intake. Again, this is all right as long as you are able to maintain a proper nutritional balance. But if you deprive yourself of basic nutritional requirements, you will very likely develop renewed back trouble because of the weakness this can produce in your muscles.

As for one-to-one contests, the racquet sports—tennis, squash, badminton, paddle ball, and even ping-pong—can be strenuous. But they certainly can be engaged in if done so prudently. If you are a tennis buff it would be wise to modify your serve so that when you reach up to hit the ball you do not excessively arch your back. You may lose some power on your serve, but you'll be able to play without the fear of re-straining your back. And, as you work on making your points on the rally, you'll become an all-round better tennis player.

Bowling, though seemingly innocuous, can be very strenuous on a weak spine (remember, until you've been at the therapeutic exercises for a sufficient time, you've got a weak spine). The bending to one side and the twisting of the spine as you release the ball can wrench your back if you're not careful. On the other hand, if your back is in good condition bowling can be beneficial. People who bowl regularly generally do not have problems because their back muscles are conditioned to the motions. But those of you who bowl only occasionally should take care.

Golf has little to recommend it from a physical therapy point of view. In addition, the game of golf seems to create more tensions than it relieves, although there are some aspects of hitting that little ball that can be tension-relieving. It certainly can't be called exercise except in the sense that going for a long walk is exercise. And even that benefit is fast losing its value as more and more golfers take to carts to get them around the links. If you can play golf without getting tense about it, by all means do.

Football, even touch football is a dangerous sport for those people with chronic back problems. The sudden twisting motions, jumping up for passes or getting blocked, can injure the back. Basketball, an excellent conditioning sport, unfortunately can cause havoc for your lower back. Arching the back as you spring upward toward the basket or landing hard on your heels with your spine extended may make you regret the moment you stepped onto the court. However, I am sensitive to the needs of people to compete, especially in team sports. So, if you approach these sports with caution and good sense, you may be able to have fun and exercise without damaging your back. Remember to warm up well before you begin anything that requires strenuous or sudden movements of your body.

Baseball, particularly softball, occupies a special place in the post-graduate heart, whether it be post-graduate from high school or college. It is a fun and social sport that does not require much effort or prior body conditioning. However, if you are not accustomed to swinging a bat on a regular basis, a mighty swing may just about tear your back muscles off the spine. Be careful; even with baseball you should be in good condition and warm up well.

There are a number of other marginal sports which fall into this category—that is, they are not particularly bad for you if you are in good condition, but they are not particularly good if you're not. The main thought I wish to convey to you with respect to sports is that you should use common sense when participating in any athletic contest. First, if you are having back pain, do not play. Make sure you are well rested, that your pain is entirely absent, and that your back is reasonably strong before you participate again. When you do play, warm up well, using your therapeutic back exercises and light calisthenics, before the competition starts. Stop when you feel your muscles fatiguing or your reflexes slowing, for this is the time when you are most likely to re-injure your back.

Except for heavy contact sports, no sports activity should be beyond your capability once you've got your back in condition, as well as the rest of you.

Sex

A great number of back-pain patients I see have profound anxiety about the effect their condition is having and will have on their sex lives. Interestingly enough, my women patients are usually much more direct and frank about discussing this problem, whereas men will hedge and talk around it. But a problem it obviously is, since the back plays such an important role in both the conventional and acrobatic maneuvers of sexual intercourse.

Now, I certainly do not intend to make this section a sex guide. Dr. Reuben presumably explained all you wanted to know about sex and were afraid to ask in his popular book. What I wish to do is indicate how sexual activities can be carried out without further straining an already weak back or in spite of the fact that one or both partners has back pain. As you probably are aware from personal experience, sexual urges have been known to conquer all sorts of obstacles, including back pain. I would like to suggest ways which will make the fulfillment of that urge less painful.

In all seriousness, back pain has been known to make men impotent and women frigid. In these instances there is nothing physiologically wrong with the individuals—they are merely psychologically reacting to pain or to the threat of pain.

One of my patients recently confided to me that for three months after being discharged from the hospital, where he had been treated for a slipped disc with bed rest and traction, he was still fearful of having intercourse with his wife. Indeed, so fearful was he of provoking a recurrence of his disc pain that he was literally unable to have an erection. This obviously created emotional strains and tensions with his wife, as well as with himself. His fears were real—they were not imaginary, they were not unfounded.

I urged him to go home immediately, explain his problem to his wife, and enlist her help. Fortunately, she was sympathetic and willing, even though he at first was reluctant to try the position I recommended. But with the encouragement of his wife he finally tried, and soon was able to return to normal relations.

Similarly, a woman patient complained of having turned frigid—the whole idea of resuming sexual relations with her husband after she had been treated for a disc problem terrified her. When she did have sexual intercourse she lived in terror and made the entire experience disagreeable for both her husband and herself.

Neither of these situations need occur just because you have back pain. In sexual relations, as with every other physical activity, the principles of sensible back care still hold true. If someone is in severe pain from a bad back strain or a red-hot disc, it is better for him or her to abstain from sex, at least for a few days or until the pain subsides. Then, when relations are resumed, the partner with the bad back should not attempt to lie on top of the other partner. This increases pressure on the lumbar spine and can aggravate the condition, and what may have started as a sublime and tender desire may end in painful shame.

Having intercourse while lying on your side and facing your partner is also difficult. For satisfactory copulation in this position the woman must place her lower leg under her mate's waist. If either she or her mate have back pain, this will make it worse.

The best position in which to have intercourse during back pain is the "spoon position." In this position the woman lies on her side with her knees flexed, while the man lies behind her, facing her back and fitting his body to her contours. In this way both backs are fairly relaxed, yet there is ample freedom of movement. Most of the back movement involved in this position is flexion movement, which is usually comfortable and not pain-aggravating.

In general, sexual partners who have back problems should be leery of trying out the more acrobatic positions often described in sex manuals as conducive to variety. Variety is fine, if you can handle it, but most mature and experienced people have long ago learned that variety of position is not the essence of good sex—love, tenderness, and the desire to please are. The sensible person with back pain can have as active a sexual life as he or she desires so long as a sympathetic and understanding partner goes along with it. But it's not enough to accept your pain and the limitations it places on you. The sensible person will eliminate the pain through therapy and by so doing will enlarge and expand his or her sexual horizons.

Sexual relations, using sensible positions, can be therapeutic. When I was an intern I frequently played basketball as a form of recreation and exercise. One of my fellow interns, a very active young man, twisted his back during a game and hobbled off the court in considerable pain. He knew he should have gone right to bed, but there was a party that night that he felt he just couldn't miss, especially because it was his girl friend who was giving it. He dragged himself to the party and lay down in a quiet corner where everyone brought him whatever he needed in the form of food, drink and sympathy. He was obviously having a pretty good time in spite of his pain and incapacity. Since the party was at his girl's apartment he decided to linger for a while after everyone else left. He assured us that he would be able to get back to the hospital under his own power.

The next morning I was amazed to see him on his feet making surgical rounds. He looked comfortable, his back was straight, and he was walking without any difficulty. I went over to him and asked him how he could account for this dramatic turnabout in his condition. He looked at me, smiled, and gave me a wink. "Worked it out last night," he said cryptically.

The gentle push-pull thrusts of the pelvis during sexual intercourse not only contribute to sexual pleasure and fulfillment, they can also be good therapy for an ailing back if done properly. Keep that in mind next time you are reluctant about having sex because of your fear of back pain.

21.

Conclusion

Now at the end of my story, I hope you have learned many things. I hope you have learned about the mechanics of your back, about the nature of and possible reasons for your back pain, about the effects of an under-exercised and tension-filled way of life on your back, about what your doctor can do to help you. Most importantly, I hope you've learned about what you must do to contend with and overcome your back pain.

In concluding this book I must refer back to the Foreword. There I said that, as a practicing orthopaedic surgeon, I know the great majority of you need not continue to endure the pain and wretchedness your back subjects you to. I said that most of your problems are due to ignorance and mismanagement, and that if you were aware of the most common causes of back pain and how to overcome them, you would be able to embark on the road to a happy, pain-free life.

This book is a guide to that road. It is designed to acquaint you with your back and its pain. I have tried to write about the back straightforwardly, even though at times it might have seemed complicated. I have tried to avoid fancy or clever prose, because as Shakespeare said in *Richard III*, "An honest tale spreads best being simply told." I have tried to avoid being too technical about a very technical subject, yet I have tried to cover all the bases of back pain.

The book is not intended to replace your doctor. But if you've read it carefully it should make your doctor's—and your—job much easier as you go about dealing with the problem of solving your back pain.

If nothing else I hope I've gotten the point across to you that, when all is said and done, it is no one else but you who is going to control and, hopefully, eliminate your back pain.

Our modern way of life with all its luxuries, fast-food services, and instant gratifications, can easily make you forget that you are responsible for the health of your body. You cannot push a button and get your body or your back well. You cannot be physically fit without working at it. I have stressed the importance of knowledge and understanding the mechanics of your back, of the interrelationship of the anatomical structures of the spine and particularly the need for strong and reliable muscles. The therapeutic exercise program has worked for me and for thousands of my patients. You can make it work for you too.

You can do it too. Perhaps in the process you will find revived in yourself not only a healthy back, but a renewed appreciation for some of the excellent and beneficial values that once sustained us, but which many of us have forgotten in the rush of time and progress. By this I mean especially the value of pride in self-improvement and in conquering the forces that, every day, seek to make you less, rather than more, of a person.

I hope this book will be of aid to you in restoring both your back and your pride in yourself. As you embark on these programs, I wish you well.

Index

Abdomen, 54, 60, 68, 152
Abdominal muscles, 30–31, 33
  exercises for, 181, 187–88,
    189–90
  and girdles, 203
  laxness of, 93, 98
  and trauma, 79–80
Abductor muscles, 34
Acetabula, 25–26
Adductor muscles, 34
Adrenal glands, 58, 142, 165
Afferent (receptor) nerves, 40–
    41, 43
Aging process, 59–60, 196–203,
    174
  and discs, 21–32, 59, 134–35,
    193
Anaesthetics, 71, 82
Analgesics, 84, 86
Anatomy (Gray's), 18
Anatomy:
  basic spinal, 17–26, 27–36,
    37–46, 51–53
  defective, 54, 56, 120–24
  evolution of, 4–5, 18, 35
  strengthening, 13–15
Angina pectoris, 80
Annulus fibrosus, 29, 104, 135
  and slipped disc, 108–9, 111
Antibiotics, 125–27
Appetite, loss of, 126, 127, 131
Arteries, 59, 143–44
Arteriosclerosis, 59, 67, 143
Arthritis, 57–58, 134–38
  diagnosis, 67, 72, 74, 133
  and disc disease, 110, 118,
    135, 193

gouty, 58, 137–38
and muscle atrophy, 66
rheumatoid, 57–58, 82, 137,
    138, 140
septic, 57
See also Osteoarthritis
Articular facets, 21, 106, 123
  asymmetric, 118, 122
Aspirin, 81–82
Autonomic nervous system, 40,
    157

Bacteria, 56, 126, 128
Barr, J. C., 103
Bed rest, 112–13, 128, 136
  contraindications, 11, 149
  after trauma, 81–82, 84
Biopsy, 126, 128, 131, 132
Bladder, 25, 110, 121
Bleeding, internal, 83
Blood:
  circulation. *See* Circulatory
    system
  clotting, 143–44
  and endocrine system, 140–
    41, 142
  and infections, 17, 126, 128
  tests, 72, 113, 131, 138, 142–
    43
Blood count, 72
Blood pressure, 165
Blood sugar, 72
Blood urea nitrogen, 72, 138
Blood vessels, 4, 13, 56, 95
  arteries, 59, 143–44

215